do
Eibhlín Uí Chatháin agus a h-iníon Eibhlín
agus i ndíl chuimhne ar
Mhártan Ó Catháin (a fuair bás 1965)

MÉINÍ THE BLASKET NURSE

LESLIE MATSON

MERCIER PRESS

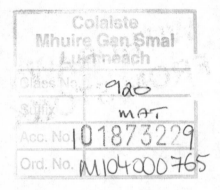
First published in 1996 by
MERCIER PRESS

Trade enquiries to CMD DISTRIBUTION,
55a Spruce Avenue,
Stillorgan Industrial Park,
Blackrock, County Dublin
Tel: (01) 294 2560; Fax: (01) 294 2564

© Leslie Matson 1995

ISBN 1 85635 133 5
10 9 8 7 6

A CIP record for this title is available
from the British Library

Cover design by Niamh Sharkey from
author's photographs
Set by Richard Parfrey
Printed in Ireland by Colour Books,
Baldoyle Industrial Estate, Dublin 13

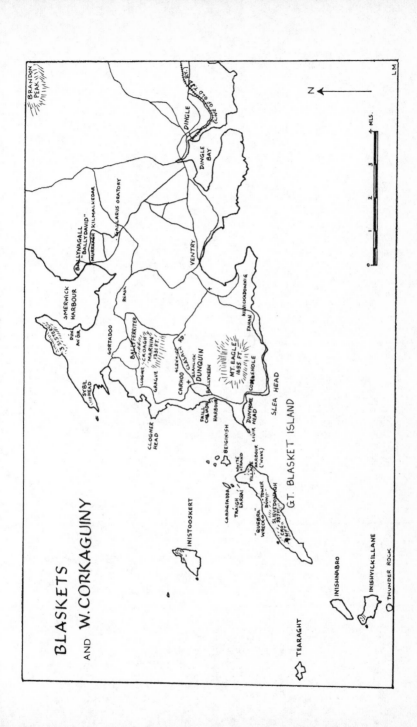

BLASKETS
AND W.CORKAGUINY

N

0 1 2 3 4 MLS.

TEARAGHT

INISHNABRO

INISHVICKILLANE
THUNDER ROCK

INISTOOSKERT

CARRAIGFADDA
TRÁIGH
EARRAÍ
"QUEBRA"
WRECK
"TOWER" DÚNPÉ
WHITE ISLAND
VILLAGE
HARBOUR ("HA")
SLIEVEDONAGH 957FT.
GT. BLASKET ISLAND

BEIGINISH

CLOGHER HEAD

FAILL CHLOGHAIR
HARBOUR

DUNMORE
LIÚIR HEAD
DUNQUIN
SLEA HEAD
COUMEENOLE

SYBIL HEAD
THREE SISTERS

SMERWICK HARBOUR
Dún An Óir

GORTADOO

BALLYFERRITER
CROAGH MARHIN 1351FT.
LISTRIM
GRAIGUE
CARHOO
CLASACH RD.
GLENLOUGH
BALLYNICK
BALLYKEEN

MT EAGLE 1695 FT.

BRANDON PEAK

BALLYNAGALL
"BALLYDAVID"
MURREAGH KILMALKEDAR
GALLARUS ORATORY

RIASK

BRASK

VENTRY

KILVICKADOWNIG
FAHAN

DINGLE BAY

DINGLE
CÉIDE OÍGH

LM

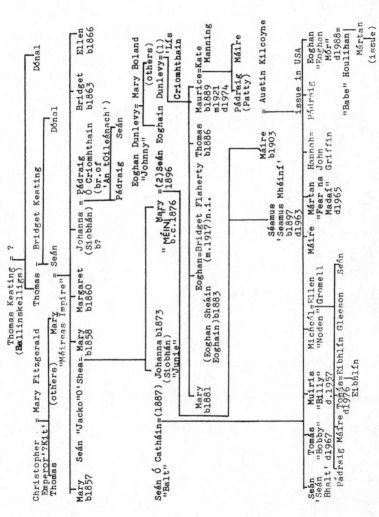

MÉINÍ'S FAMILY
(main details only)

CONTENTS

FOREWORD

This is the life-story of a remarkable woman, whose friendship I was privileged to share when she was old and I was young. Born in the United States of Kerry parents, she was brought back to her grandparents' house in Dunquin in her earliest years. She returned to the land of her birth for a short spell in her teens but at the age of nineteen she came home again, very soon crossing to the Blasket island where she lived as nurse and midwife for thirty-six years, married to a widower very much older than herself.

The notes I took down from Méiní and her friends in the late 1950s and early 1960s stimulated an interest in the life of Dunquin and the Blaskets which has remained with me ever since. The notes remained, frequently read but otherwise unused, until eventually I was able to transmute them into this story. Of course, I was helped in this by many other writings. In Tomás Ó Criomhthain's *Allagar na hInise* (Island Cross-Talk), for example, Méiní and her husband appear as Nell and Tadhg the Joker. We meet them in Robin Flower's *The Western Island*, and there is an account of her life (a highly selective or, possibly, selected one) which she gave to Mícheál Ó Gaoithín, Peig Sayers's son, for the Irish Folklore Commission.

This tale makes no claim to scholarship, since in the fields of Irish and of folklore studies I have no qualifications. Nevertheless, I have stated nothing as fact which I do not believe on good authority to be true. For this reason, I hope it will offend no real scholar, and that the general reader will find something of interest in the story of this memorable woman.

Readers of Irish will immediately note certain inconsistencies in spelling. For place-names in English I have used the versions favoured by An Seabhach in *Triocha-Céad Chorca Dhuibhne*. I have put personal names into forms or equivalents more easily pronounceable for readers of English, with one or two exceptions. Tomás Ó Criomhthain's name is so familiar in this (possibly incorrect) form, that it would be somewhat perverse to abandon it. Mícheál Ó Gaoithín would be reluctant to have his name translated, and for him Mike Pheig and the *File* (poet) are also used. I have also retained many of the patronymic forms when in general use. How much more attractive is, for example, Muirisín Mharas Mhuiris, and how much more full of social history, than Little Maurice Maurice Maurice?

I am grateful to many people whose help was freely given in recording information about Méiní. Writings about West Kerry and the Blaskets are numerous and the help they have given has been acknowledged in the text. Among those who supplied me with information and hospitality, for which I am most grateful, are the following:

Professor Bo Almqvist
Eibhlín, Bean Uí Chatháin
Bídí, Bean Uí Chatháin (Bríd Mharas Mhuiris)
Eoghan Ó Catháin (Eoghan Mór) (ná maireann)
Mártan Ó Catháin (ná maireann)
Mártan and Betty Ó Catháin
Seán Mharas Mhuiris Ó Catháin (ná maireann)
Seán Pheats Tom Ó Ceárnaigh
Molly O'Connor
An Dr Seosamh Ó Dálaigh (ná maireann)
Mícheál Ó Dubhshláine, OS
Pádraig Ó Duinnlé
Muiris Mhaidhc Léan Ó Gaoithín
Seán Mhaidhc Léan Ó Gaoithín
John Larry Ó Cíobháin (ná maireann)
The late Muiris Kavanagh (Kruger)
The late Séamus 'Twoee' Kavanagh

Bid Ní Lúing
Máire, Bean Uí Lúing
Walter McGrath
Eibhlín, Bean Uí Mhaolcatha
Mícheál Mistéal
Lisa, Bean Uí Mhistéal (ná maireann)
Mícheál de Mórdha
Ríonach Uí Ógáin
Máirín, Bean Mhic Shíthigh (ná maireann)
Frank Mac Síthigh
Ray Stagles

I am particularly indebted to Mícheál de Mórdha for his encouragement in the publication of this book and to the O'Brien Press for permission to use the photograph of Méiní and Gobnait Kennedy which first appeared in Ray and Joan Stagles's *The Blasket Islands* (second edition).

I am grateful to Professor Bo Almqvist of the Department of Irish Folklore, UCD, for permission to quote from the account of Méiní's life which she gave to Mícheál Ó Gaoithín while he was a collector for the Irish Folklore Commission.

The dedication records my special debt to Eibhlín Uí Chatháin and her daughter, also Eibhlín, who not only have been most hospitable to me in Dunquin, but have lovingly maintained Méiní's house on the cliff-top. Eibhlín's husband Tomás looked after Méiní in her last illness, and died tragically in 1976.

With deep respect I dedicate this book also to the memory of my friend Mártan Ó Catháin, who first introduced me to his aunt and cared for her literally to the last minute of his own life.

Ar dheis Dé go raibh a n-anamacha dílse uaisle.

Cork/Waterford/Millstreet, 1995

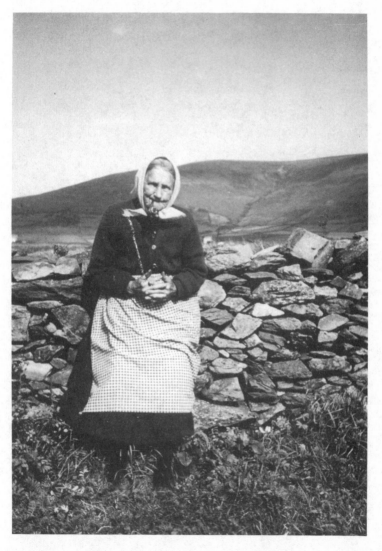

Méiní, aged 84, with her beloved pipe

1
—

TWILIGHT

The table at which I sat was made of rough deal planks, and the *súgán* of my chair was encrusted with grime. On the far side of the fire stood a crudely made three-legged stool – it alone could remain steady on the uneven earthen floor. Through the window beside me nothing could now be seen of Eagle Mountain. Across the room the other tiny window had gathered the last of the light as the early autumn sun had settled down behind the fluted cone of the Tearaght; it had now become a mirror, and reflected back the flame of the candle standing on the table before me. This was the only light, for the soft turf from the top of the bog, the *móin stuaicín*, had been placed over the glowing ashes of the hard dark sods which had boiled the kettle and the fish. Tomorrow, the soft turf which had tamed the flame and nursed it overnight would be blown into life again and a few hard lumps added to bring the kettle, hanging on its adjustable iron hook, quickly to the boil for the breakfast tea. Clamped to the wall was a crude wooden shelf. The glare of the candle cut off whatever lay beyond. The half-door was closed top and bottom, but a cool breeze sweeping down the high ground to the east in the direction of the sea had no difficulty in finding its way through. I knew that out there lay the dog, tethered to an old iron bedstead in the tiny stepping-stoned garden, to keep him from the sheep on the common land of Ballykeen.

No need to pierce the candleglow. At the side of the room farthest from the fire I knew that two old iron beds stood end to end. In one of them the posts at the foot and at the head leaned crazily towards each other, such was the curve in the frame of its base, dipping down almost to touch the cracked old chamber-pot beneath. The other bed was sturdier but equally old. I could hear murmuring, a purring of English phrases, repeated again and again. I knew that in this bed, her back to the sea, Méiní sat as straight upright as her tired old back would allow her. Her gnarled hands would be held before her face, their fingers furrowed by deep ridges, and streaked by handling the burning turf or from pushing the tobacco down into the *dúidín* when it was burning well.

'Holy Mary, Mother o' God' . . . I could just make out the syllables; an occasional groan answered a passing thought of sadness or a twinge in her stiff back. The old skirt would be on her still, and the check apron which she lifted to wipe her mouth before she gave you a kiss. An extra cardigan kept her warm for the night; the scarf which sometimes fell around her neck during the day was now drawn up over her head, almost covering her face.

Another groan, and I realised that the prayers had stopped. I waited. If the creaking of the bed told me she was settling down there would be no more stories tonight, no laughter about old Dr Hudson or Peggy 'Flint' or Nell Mhicil, no tales of the priest's cabbages or of Tí Mhóire. The drone of the prayers had now been replaced by the muted pulse of regular breathing. Time for me to go. No sound yet of Martin's crutches on the flags, returning to sleep in the other bed after chatting to Mícheál down at Béal Átha. '*Codladh sámh*, sleep tight!' – I said it very gently as I made

18

for the door, but there was no answering farewell. Tomorrow I would call again and her eyes would sparkle as she fiddled with her pipe. 'Italy, *a bhuachaill*,' (for that was as near as she could get to my strange name), 'I've another story for you! The *File* wanted to get it but I kept it for you.' That was to be another day. I closed the door behind me and set off through the fields to the road which led north through Ballinaraha to Kruger's. Another evening with Méiní was over.

2

TRAVELS AND TRAGEDIES

Some time towards the middle of the nineteenth century, Bridget Keating arrived in Gleann Mór beside which the old road from Ventry drops down from the Clasach to the cross at Dunquin, the most westerly parish in Europe, the next one to America. Her two sons, Seán and Dónal were with her but she was in a sorry plight. Her husband Tom had collapsed and died on the road not far from his abandoned home at Tobar Mhíchíl (St Michael's Well) near Ballinskelligs, on the southern Kerry peninsula of Iveragh. Of a heart attack, it was said, but it was a broken heart already, for he had been driven by the landlord from the land he had inherited.

Tom's father, also Tom, had been comparatively prosperous, with the grass for twenty cows, and after his death the farm had been divided between Tom and his brother Dónal, with grass for ten cows each. Dónal had a taste for drink and did not long retain possession of his share. Tom worked hard on his smallholding, which he hoped to pass on in his turn to one of his sons. A vain hope, as it transpired, for the greed of the landlord dashed his plans and he had no alternative but to set out to find work and a home somewhere else. Links between the southern peninsula and the Dingle area were strong because of the fishing trade, but it seems strange that the little family should have set out for such an impoverished part of the country. There may have been a forgotten family connection. Now Tom lay buried, back again at Tobar Mhíchíl.

Bridget, also a Keating by birth, earned the sympathy of the people of the valley of Gleann Mór for her sad plight, and a cottage was soon found for her. No doubt she did odd jobs about the neighbourhood to support her family, herding cows, working in the fields and spinning the wool from the mountain sheep. When the two brothers, Seán and Dónal were old enough, they set about earning a living for themselves from fishing, first of all helping to form crews with the local fishermen. At that time, the canvas-covered *naomhóga* had not yet been introduced into the area and bigger boats were used even though they were vulnerable to confiscation. Gleann Mór was proving inconvenient because the landing place at Faill Chliadh was a mile or so from their home and time was wasted in getting there. The masters of the boats had to be able to take to the sea at short notice and potential crews had to be on the spot.

In Ballykeen, as close as it was possible to get, stood an empty house which had been used during the famine to dispense soup. This distribution had stopped a few years before but the old boiler was still there. The house was somewhat different from the usual type, having a big window on the landward side through which the soup had been handed out. It was not a very cosy house, for in the evenings the cold off-shore winds easily found a way through, but Dónal and Seán were glad to take it over, and they were soon joined by their mother from Gleann Mór. Within a few years she died and was buried in Ballinahow. Dónal eventually left, joined the Kerry Militia, and died many years later in Chicago. The way was open for Seán to bring a wife into the house.

Within the same townland of Ballykeen stood a house

21

which was recorded in 1850 as belonging to Thomas Emperor. With a name as unusual and striking as that it was only natural that various explanations of his origin should be put forward, one being that he was a Spaniard whose forebears arrived at the time of the Smerwick massacre of November 1580. In fact, the Emperor family held land near Rockchapel on the Cork-Limerick border and some is still in their name. The modern representatives of the family have no idea of their origin, apart from vague references to Spain and France, and the most likely explanation is that they came from England. Kit Emperor, for thus he seems to have been called since his second name was Christopher, is first heard of as running a mill in Ballincota, near Ventry, but there is evidence that the family had connections with the village of Boolteens near Castlemaine at the head of the peninsula. By trade he was a carpenter, and by all accounts a very good one, and he ran the mill at Ballincota with at least one other brother.

Some time around 1830, Kit met and married Mary Fitzgerald, also living in Ventry parish. Although the house in Dunquin was in his name, or possibly that of a son, Thomas, in 1850, it is likely that by then his marriage had broken down. In fact he may never have lived in Dunquin himself and his wife may have moved there to be nearer to her sister Bridget who was married to a Malone from Coomenoule. He sailed for America leaving his wife, as far as we know, with one son and pregnant with a daughter Máire, pet-named Méireas. It is almost certain that he never returned to Ireland

In due course, sometime around the year 1855, Seán Keating married Méireas 'Ímpire', and brought her to his home. They had six children, by their granddaughter's reckoning, which included Siobhán (Johanna), Máire and Ellen (Nora) who was baptised in 1866. Siobhán married Paddy Ó Criomhthain, brother of the Islandman, Tomás Ó Criomhthain, and went to live on the Great Blasket where she had two sons before dying at an early age. These two boys settled in the States and will make a brief reappearance in our story. For a short time their father lived there too, returning to spend most of his later life on the Blaskets.

Máire Keating, around the year 1872, married Seán Jacko O'Shea, who lived a few miles from Dunquin in Baile Eaglaise, about a mile northwest of Ballyferriter. Jacko's father had died, and his mother and two aunts, Máire and Cáit, had gone to live in Chicopee, near Springfield, Massachusetts. Apparently they were satisfied with their life there, and in the year 1875 or thereabouts they persuaded Jacko to leave his home farm and bring his young wife Máire and their daughter Junie, who had been born in 1873, to live in Chicopee also. Shortly after their arrival, a second child was born, who, by her own account was baptised at Chicopee Falls by Fr Timothy Healy, on 27 April, probably in the year 1876. They called her Máire after her mother and grandmother, but to the end of her life everyone knew her as Méiní.

Within two years Jacko died, and was buried in what Méiní referred to as a lonely cemetery in Chicopee Falls. It seems unlikely that his mother and both his aunts would have died in this short period also, but Máire seems to have been left alone with Junie and the infant Méiní then about two years of age. She found it very difficult to cope with the many demands on her, since she had to work outside the home to maintain her little family. She sent word to her parents, and without delay Seán and Méireas crossed the Atlantic to help her. On arrival in Chicopee, Seán acquired a house of his own and was soon in employment. Máire and her children moved in with them.

After two years, Seán's health was beginning to fail and the doctor ordered him back to Ireland. Máire decided to part from Méiní, who returned with Seán and Méireas to Dunquin.

Méiní's account of this journey, given in her old age, no

doubt echoed phrases remembered from her grandparents. For three months they were on the bosom of the sea, one day forward, one day backward. Eventually, Ireland was reached, and soon Dunquin.

Máire continued her work for a year or two, but, deprived of her parents' support, she found it impossible to continue, and in her turn she crossed the sea with her elder daughter.

At this time, Seán Keating was making his living as a weaver and Máire joined him at his work. Indeed, she may have been helping him before her marriage to Jacko. Seán had been a fisherman to begin with but he never liked the life and sought out other means of making ends meet. A man called Sexton who lived at Poulgorm in Ventry parish had a wide reputation as a fine weaver, and Seán persuaded Méireas that he should go and work for Sexton to learn the trade. After a year or two he was sufficiently expert to set up his own loom in Dunquin and to pass on his skills to Máire. There was little cash to spare, and Méiní often wondered how her mother's dowry had been saved up.

In spite of the rigours of the journey home and the strain consequent on the death of her young husband, Máire had arrived in very good health and with a prosperous appearance. This fact made an impression on her parents and even more so on her younger sister Nora. The latter persuaded her father to cross the Atlantic with her so that she could settle in the United States. The fact that she was suffering from some disease, most likely a chest complaint, convinced the parents that a change of climate might do her good and they agreed to her request. Their journey had a strange sequel.

When Seán arrived in New York with Nora, he met a man from Dingle, a Mr White, who said that he knew of another Irishman who would employ him in a cotton mill. When he was introduced, the potential employer turned out to be none other than Thomas Emperor, his own wife's fugitive father, whom she herself had never seen and who was now in his seventies. Emperor's reaction was not what would have been expected in the circumstances: he welcomed his son-in-law warmly. By this stage he was living with his third wife. His first American wife had been killed in a storm, leaving him two sons. He gave instructions that Nora, who was, after all, his own grandchild, was to be well looked after.

Seán Keating worked as a foreman for Emperor at his mill, but his loyalty was under strain and he contacted his mother-in-law, Mary Fitzgerald, Emperor's lawful wife, suggesting that she come to claim her rights. Having spent some years in England when it was clear that her errant spouse was not going to return, she was now living back again in Kerry, possibly at Ballincota. She decided to press her case and, armed with her marriage certificate and references from the parish priest, she set off for America. Emperor resisted her demands in the courts and she apparently gained very little for her pains. Strangely enough, it appears that the litigation had no effect on Emperor's relationship with his granddaughter Nora who, as her niece Méiní maintained, continued as a member of his household and lacked for nothing until the day of her death.

The hapless Mary Fitzgerald returned to Ireland and presumably Seán Keating went with her. He made at least two further trips to the States, possibly to visit his daughter or to supplement his meagre income. The hot climate did not suit him and aggravated some medical condition from which he suffered. As he moved through middle age he settled down to his weaving, helped by Máire, and supplied the people of Dunquin and district. He may have worked occasionally for the Blasket islanders, as his daughter Siobhán lived there after her marriage, but in general they would have patronised Eoghan Bán O'Connor, who lived and worked in the buildings which had been the old Protestant Mission School.

3

CHILDHOOD

The young widow Máire settled down to help her father with his weaving and later developed, as we shall see, another source of income. Now that she was safely home she could measure the extent of her loss. Her young husband lay dead and buried thousands of miles away, her two young girls unprovided for. But they were growing up fast and the sight of them running about her feet as she worked at the loom helped her to bear her sorrow. Junie was her favourite, the child of her first passion. As she grew older, Méiní felt this strongly, and reacted uneasily to her mother's favouritism.

At the age of eight she was taken by Máire to the national school to join Junie there. The teacher Seán Ó Dálaigh was a remarkable man who under the pen-name of 'Common Noun' was to write books about local life and customs. His father had been tragically killed in a fire in Ballykeen about fourteen years before and he was now in the final years of his training, having been taken on as a monitor or student teacher to his uncle Dónal Moriarty at an earlier stage. He and Michael Manning of Ballyferriter were among the first teachers to gain an official honours certificate recognising their capacity to teach the Irish language, though at the time such teaching was restricted to before and after school hours and to classes above fourth standard. A local man whose own family was to make a big contribution to Irish studies, Ó Dálaigh was nevertheless cast in a traditional mould and Méiní recalled his strap and pointer without enthusiasm.

The elder generation at this time, although they spoke Irish among themselves, looked on the acquisition of English as a necessity for survival at home and abroad. For this reason, in many families children were forced to speak English as soon as they were able, and frequently punished if they spoke Irish. By the time that she returned from the United States as an infant, Méiní was already able to speak some words of English. Máire continued to speak it to both her children as a matter of course and taught them their prayers in it. Accordingly, when Méiní went to school, she talked English much better than most of her classmates. In fact, she took a pride in claiming that the senior children used to gather around her to hear her talk. Naturally enough, when she mixed with her friends outside school she spoke Irish only, as it came more naturally to them, but she was wary of pretending to a knowledge of it at home. On one occasion her grandmother Méireas asked her in Irish, '*An bhfacaís an t-asal?* – Did you see the donkey?' but she was not to be caught out. Putting on as innocent a face as she could manage she replied, 'And what does that mean, Grandmother?' When she told that story three-quarters of a century later she could not hold back a warm chuckle.

We do not know precisely why Méiní left school, because she has given two separate accounts of it. There seems little doubt that she was a poor scholar with a strong taste for conviviality and it may have been true that Ó Dálaigh suggested to her mother that by age twelve she had got all she could from the school. Her other more circumstantial explanation is more likely to be true, as it contains details which she would have been unlikely to want to invent. Seán

Ó Dálaigh went to Dublin for the final stages of his training around about 1885 and he was replaced by a temporary teacher from Kilkenny, a Mr Gleeson, who charged fees, as sometimes happened in those days. Máire felt that these were too high and Méireas appealed to Fr Egan, the parish priest. He was unwilling to go against the teacher and as a result Méiní was taken away, as were a few other pupils. She was now only about ten years of age and her mother attempted to get her into the Protestant mission school at Ballinaraha. This was known as *Tigh Fallon* but Méiní called it Fitzgerald's school, possibly because a Maurice Fitzgerald had taught there in 1831. She was not accepted and her schooling came to an abrupt end.

Her sister Junie had, as Méiní recounts, an eye for the lads, and about the time that the latter left school, she married Seán Keane in January 1887 when she was almost exactly fourteen years of age. The story that she was enticed into this marriage by the offer of a bag of sweets is probably apocryphal and is explicable as an invention founded on her unusually tender age. She settled down to bring up a large family a few hundred yards from her home near the site of the old mill where the Dunquin river enters the sea at Béal Átha.

When Méiní was about ten there was a further upheaval as, just below their house, work was being done on the approaches to the old landing place at Faill Chliadh, to make it more accessible to the top of the cliff. Méiní remembered a man called George Coller (more likely Collier, a name recorded in Dingle), who lodged in their cottage for the year he was working there. During this period they moved up to the little chapel-of-ease which stood beside them on the exact spot where the house in which Méiní passed her later years still stands. There was still a roof on the little chapel which had been out of use since the building in 1857 of the existing church in Ballintemple. Local memory associates it with a priest who abandoned his faith and married a minister's daughter. It may have been that Denis Brasbie celebrated Mass there before his conversion to Protestantism in 1844 which was publicly announced in a provocative way, causing understandable offence to the Catholic people in Dingle and necessitating military intervention to ensure public order.

In school, Méiní's special friends had been Peg Sheehy, Peg Keane, sister to the man who married Junie, and Kate Moriarty. The friendship with Kate was particularly strong and they lived close to each other. When they left school both girls had to work very hard. This they did together when it was possible. Since there was no boy in the family and Seán Keating was middle-aged and fully occupied with his weaving, a great deal of outside work fell on Méiní in her early teens. When the tide threw up large quantities of seaweed down by Béal Átha it was Méiní's job to wade out and collect it in creels, dripping wet and almost heavy enough to break her back. She had to carry it up to the tiny patch of land to spread it out where the staple diet of potatoes was grown. In the summer the potato-pit had to be dug and filled. Some expeditions would take her up to the slopes of Mount Eagle and Coomaleague Hill, or, farther north, climbing beyond Ferriter's Quarter (Carhoo) to Croagh Marhin, the Diarmuid's Bed of the local folklore. She would bring back loads of the gnarled branches of the dead furze to supplement the turf firing and to keep alive the open fire which was the only source of heat and on which all the cooking had to be done.

Already in her teens Méiní found herself an aunt, for Junie was starting her large family, of whom nine survived. Her husband Seán, nicknamed Balt, was a son of 'Muiris na Tinte' (Maurice of the Tent). The latter had been born, as had his two brothers Pat and Tom, in the island of Inishtooskert, their family being liable to be cut off by bad weather for weeks at a time. His first move was to the Great Blasket where he married Mary Counihan from Ballinvoher parish, near Annascaul. Seán's brother was known as Mikil Chuainí, presumably because of his mother's surname, and he and his wife Nell were parents of the line of musicians who bore the nickname 'Casht'. Maurice and Mary moved from the Blaskets to settle in Béal Átha near where Nell Boland had built her mill earlier in the century and the temporary shelter which Maurice first built may have earned him his title.

While Méiní was working hard outside, her mother was developing another source of income. Willie Long from Ballyferriter was an enterprising merchant whose daughter taught in Dunquin school, and when taking her to school in his horse-drawn trap he used to carry ten-stone bags of flour and Indian meal. Máire acted as his agent to sell these to the Blasket islanders. A big-boned woman, she had no difficulty in handling the heavy bags and had earned a reputation for keeping businesslike accounts. The flour and meal would be transferred from Willie Long's trap on to the back of her father's white donkey – *asal bán Chéitinn* is still referred to by old people – and brought down prior to 1903 to the old harbour under Faill Chliadh for transport to the Blaskets. Coming back from the harbour, Máire would often bring mackerel caught by the islanders on their way across. Instead of cleaning them in the sea-water before climbing the steep slope, or dipping them in a bucket of water, she used to wipe them with a damp cloth, an eccentricity which did not escape her neighbours. She kept a cow which was well looked after and carefully housed, and she had a reputation for hospitality. Peig Sayers's poet son Mike has described how delighted Máire was to see his mother when she called on her trips back from the island, and how she would press her to stay to have a cup of tea with them.

It was a busy household in which Méiní grew into her teens, with customers calling for her grandfather and Máire.

Her grandmother had occasional callers too, for Méireas was possessed of a singular gift. Not only was she knowledgeable about herbs and traditional remedies but she had the reputation of having the cure for *craosghalar* (thrush), a painful fungal infection of the throat. This cure was traditionally exercised only by those who had never seen their own father and Méireas claimed this to be true in her case. Her great-grandson Martin Keane, who died in 1965, remembered that Méireas's treatment had to be carried out three mornings in a row and that the patient had to be with her before nine o'clock. Her treatment was to breathe sharply into the mouth of the patient – usually a child – while he or she was still fasting.

Mícheál Ó Gaoithín gives an account of such a visit about the year 1912 when he was nine and Méireas approximately eighty-five. The old woman told Peig first of all that if she had known of her son's illness before they left the island she could have saved her the journey by passing on a guaranteed cure. This involved forcing a gander to breathe down the boy's infected throat – a cure which would hardly have been welcomed by the patient even if a gander could have been found on the Blaskets at that time. On this occasion, Peig and Mike were going to spend a few days with her people in Baile Bhiocáire under Eagle Mountain, and Méireas gave instructions to bring the boy down fasting the next morning. Three days in a row this was done but Mike does not record whether the cure was effective.

Méiní gives one more glimpse into her early teenage years which displays a touch of harmless vanity and illustrates the poverty of her surroundings. Seán and Méireas had gone into Dingle to meet the early train, leaving Méiní in bed in the cottage. Poking around on the shelves and in the little cupboard as children will when left alone, she found a bottle of oil which her grandfather kept for putting on the whetstone when sharpening his razor. 'I caught the bottle,' she related seventy years later, 'and I poured it on my head. My hair was white at the time. When they came back there was nothing to be seen but the hair all smeared.' Méireas got a cauldron of hot water to wash the hair, but to no avail for it was matted hopelessly. The culprit was sent out into the sun to see if the oil residue would melt, but it was soon clear that there was nothing for it but to cut off the hair. 'My lovely curls would have to be cut off, every bit of them.' Méireas was sad in her fury but Méiní was broken-hearted. 'My curls never came back again, nor my nice fair hair.'

Her friendship with Kate Moriarty was the closest one of her life and from time to time Méiní used to sleep at her house on the road from Ballykeen to Ballinaraha. As the girls entered adolescence their talk would have been of the local boys, particularly the Blasket islanders who inevitably carried with them an intriguing flavour of the unknown. When she was younger Méiní used to play with Tommy 'Twoee', whose father, the original 'Twoee' Kavanagh, had been in the States during the Civil War and had earned his nickname on his return. Tommy, through the Fitzgerald sisters, was a second cousin of Máire Keating but was of an age with Méiní. At this later stage, Kate and Méiní used to go down to Faill Chliadh to meet the Blasket boys when they crossed on Sundays for Mass. Among them they had two particular favourites but Méiní's died before the romance could blossom. Kate's boyfriend – and she kept her feelings for him a secret even from Méiní at the beginning – was most likely Tomás Guiheen, nicknamed 'Plate', whom she was later to marry.

As the girls moved into their mid-teens, the idea of marriage must have been very much in their minds, but possibly because her other daughter Junie had married so young, Máire was in no hurry to arrange a match for Méiní. Her occasional flirtations did not disguise from the perceptive young lady that her situation was not an enviable one. Hard work was her lot for most of the week, collecting the seaweed, digging the potatoes or bringing back the furze and turf from the mountain. Kate was not always there to lend a hand and Junie was now preoccupied with her young family. Her natural feeling of loneliness was aggravated by the fact that every post brought to the parish news of young people – some of whom had been her schoolfriends – who now formed part of the Kerry emigrant communities around Holyoke and Springfield into which she herself had been born. Her thoughts turned to the idea of once more crossing the Atlantic, to where the far-off hills seemed daily more and more green.

4

To America and Back

When in her eighties Méiní told her story to the poet Mícheál Ó Gaoithín she omitted virtually all mention of the chapter in her life which now follows. There were other omissions at later stages which may have their origins in a desire not to re-open old sores, but it is difficult to understand this particular gap. She would have known that Mícheál had returned from his own trip to America with a feeling of failure and this may have led her to avoid related topics. Indeed, she may have been impatient to finish the story, and deliberately abridged it. Whatever the reason, my own notes make it clear that her memory of that phase of her life was just as vivid as that of other periods.

From Dunquin and from the Blaskets the young people were going. There were still many left, far too many in fact for the local small-holdings with their high proportion of boggy and mountain land to support in comfort. Over in the 'next parish', large pockets of Kerry people had been accumulating for fifty years since the famine chased them from home. This wave of Irishmen and Irishwomen, concentrated in the Boston region, were now in their sixties and seventies. Their children were American citizens but they maintained their devotion to Irish interests and culture.

They welcomed their cousins who came later, providing for them a milieu to which they could easily relate and, in many cases, the prospect of stable jobs. Not many of these young people came back, but the few who did, and the ever-welcome Christmas letters with their enclosed dollars, spoke of prosperity, comfort and a vibrant life. The young Méiní would have heard endless tales of such things around the fire in Ballykeen or in her grandfather's weaving shed. Those who called from the Blaskets on their way to Dingle or going in again, brought news of their relations too.

The news reached the Keating house in Ballykeen that 'Lís, one of the seven daughters of 'old Maurice Daly' (in J. M. Synge's phrase) from Inishvickillane had been sent the passage-money from America and was gathering herself to go, along with Peg O'Connor from the main island. Peg was a daughter of Eoghan Bán O'Connor, the island weaver, and aunt to Tomás Eoghain Bháin who was Maurice O'Sullivan's boyhood friend. Hearing this, Méiní saw her opportunity and determined to set out with 'Lís and Peg whom she would have known from Mass or dances in Dunquin.

When the three girls went to book their passage with Galvin, the White Star agent in Dingle, they discovered that they were to travel out of Cork on the *Majestic*, and would be accompanied by three lads from Letteragh over near Mount Brandon, Paddy O'Sullivan, Maurice Hannefin and Eoin Brown. The excitement of the girls was soon drowned by the realisation that in all probability they would never see their home and people again. On the island there would have been an 'American wake' on the eve of departure and then in the morning the trip across the Blasket sound to the Faill Chliadh harbour at Dunquin. At the top of Slí Whatty (a track that had been built by the Scottish coastguard Watty Hill) Méiní and her family were waiting for them. The donkey and cart was hitched up, and the young girls with at least one member of their respective families

35

set off through Gleann Luic up the sharp slope of the Clasach road. Their friends followed them on foot to 'convey' them in the traditional way, until the top of the Clasach ridge was reached and away to the south and east Ventry and Dingle Bay came into view. Peg and 'Lís took a last look at their native islands. On the Blaskets one could pick out the bright expanse of the White Strand; the houses to the south of it snuggled so closely into the hillside that one could detect their presence only by the turf smoke. Slinneán Bán where Peig Sayers was to live would be a bare field for seventeen years more.

At the Leacht the farewells were said and the little procession started to drop down the further slopes of Marhin. In a couple of hours Dingle was reached and a lodging-house was found, probably one of those run by relations of their own families. The next morning there was immense bustle at the Dingle station. The little narrow-gauge engines were puffing up and down the sidings, attaching the cattle-wagons with their protesting occupants to the couple of passenger carriages with slatted seats which sufficed for whatever travellers were making their way to Tralee. There they transferred to the mainline train which took them through Farranfore to Killarney and on through Mallow to Cork. At Farranfore Junction they would have been joined by more emigrants speaking Irish, most of them from the Iveragh peninsula along whose northern shore ran the thrilling line to Valentia. At Loo Bridge the Kenmare branch train was waiting. On the approaches to Cork the train plunged into the long tunnel and smoke and steam swirled into the carriage, startling the girls and driving them closer to their escorts. Then, suddenly, the train burst out into the light and came to a halt along the huge crescent of the Cork platform. They knew they had not reached their destination yet, which was Queenstown, nowadays again called Cobh, the outer port of Cork, but they were probably too scared and overcome even to stretch their legs. At Queenstown they went through the customs examination, then on to the little tender which took them out past Haulbowline and Spike Island between the forts of Carlisle on the east and on the west, Camden and Templebreedy. By now the *Majestic* could be clearly seen, at anchor off Roche's Point.

One can only speculate on the feelings of the girls as the tender brought them in under the lee of the massive ship. Along with its sister-ships of uniform design, the *Brittanic*, the *Germanic* and the *Teutonic*, the *Majestic* was a vessel of which the White Star line was proud, but nevertheless it catered for steerage passengers as well as its luxury travellers. It carried the 'outfits' of the steerage passengers free of charge, and its advertisements noted that its steerage rates were low. It made a trip to New York about once a month, calling at Queenstown a day after leaving Liverpool. The scale of what they were witnessing must have driven at least temporarily from the minds of the girls the islands and the cliffs at Dunquin and the little beaches sheltered under Brandon.

As young as she was, 'Lís was already a hardened sailor. In all weathers she had crossed in the *naomhóg* from the Inish to the Great Blasket and then on to Dunquin harbour. Not only that, but her nickname was *'Lís na Beannaí*, because her mother gave birth to her as the boat in which she was travelling at the time was just abreast of the rock known as An Bheannaigh or an Bheannach near the landing place for Beiginis island. The boats which 'Lís would have been used to would have been dwarfed even by the lifeboats of the huge liner on to which she and her five companions now stepped.

The poor emigrants found their bunks down in the bowels of the ship. No dancing to the ship's orchestra for them, nor promenades on deck. The bundles containing all their worldly possessions were stacked below, but now rather timidly and overawed by the sheer size of everything, they crept to the steerage railings to watch the Irish coast drift away, as they must have thought, forever. As night fell the flashing light from the Fastnet Rock winked a last farewell. Far away to the north lay the Iveragh peninsula and beyond that again the jagged spine of Corkaguiny at whose tip their island homes were found. By this time the Atlantic swell was taking its toll on the passengers. Méiní and Peg spent the next four or five days stretched out on their cramped bunks, prostrated with seasickness. Not so 'Lís – many an expedition she had made with her father, her brother Paddy Maurice and the rest of her seafaring family as they hunted the seals and the herrings around the base of Leaca Dhubhach, the Sorrowful Slope of the Great Blasket coast which had claimed so many sailors' lives. In such company to admit to seasickness was to show a weakness which the hard life of the sea could not condone, and 'Lís had long since got her sea-legs. Paddy and Maurice and Eoin were very likely as sea-hardened as she, so she was probably not without company with whom to swop tales of her island home.

Eventually, Méiní and Peg felt well enough to wander around the permitted portion of the ship with their four friends. Calmer waters had been reached and they had got used to the motion and the sickening smell of oil. Nevertheless, it was a relief to see New York harbour although they were filled with apprehension about their new life.

At this point the three lads drop out of the story, though they probably ended up somewhere in the Springfield and Holyoke area among many of their own people. The three girls were making for Chicopee Falls where Méiní herself had been baptised. Each of them had rail tickets to get them there, but as they left the Customs House Méiní discovered to her horror that her ticket was no longer in her pocket. Somewhere amidst the fuss and bustle she had dropped it and a frantic search proved vain. When they got to the station where they were to take the train, Méiní's protestations that she had already paid for the railway ticket cut little ice with the checkers – perhaps they had heard the story too often from poor emigrants. Because it was cheaper and her very limited supply of cash was running out, Méiní had no option but to do part of the journey by steamer to Hartford. The two girls were shepherded on to the train to Chicopee Falls, and Méiní tells of no further meetings with her friends.

As she sat on the platform, weeping in her loneliness, an Irish voice asked her what she wanted. 'Seán!' cried Méiní with delight, for she recognised who was speaking to her. None other than the Carroll lad from Teeravane, four or five miles from her home over towards Clogher Strand. He could not have turned up at a better time, and, brushing away her tears, she told Seán about her lost ticket. He escorted her to the boat, where she found herself sitting on deck next to three coloured men who scared her a little as they had, in her words, 'no English or Greek or Irish'. There was no cover on deck, and when nine o'clock came, the rain began to fall in sheets. Méiní could stand it no longer and she began to walk around until she found a nice room. The soaking she received had been unnecessary and the possibility that there might have been a saloon had just not crossed her mind. She found some place where she could lie down and, exhausted by the excitement, dismay and fear of the day, her desire for sleep overcame the tension of the journey and it was six o'clock when she woke again.

Eventually, Hartford Quay was reached. A cart was waiting at the quay-side which Méiní thought might have been sent for her, but there was no one with it and the captain, seeing the little Irish girl in evident perplexity, sent a boy to put her on the ferry which brought her to the station for Springfield. When she bought the ticket her purse contained, as she remembered, the equivalent of four shillings. At Springfield, she took the train to Chicopee.

Peg and 'Lís would by this time have reached that town and the result was that Méiní's relations kept watch on the trains, a ritual which must have been a familiar one to the local Irish as emigrants from home flooded in. Méiní was not to know this and on the short journey she gazed anxiously out the window until Chicopee was reached. As she alighted, Máire O'Shea, her own namesake and a sister of her father, threw her arms about her in welcome. She had brought along two hefty Irish lads in case there was anything to be carried though she knew that it was unlikely. They were Paddy and Seán Ó Criomhthain, in all probability her own first cousins, sons of her deceased aunt Siobhán Keating and of Paddy Ó Criomhthain, and nephews of the Islandman. Since they had left Ireland they had acquired plenty of American slang and their manners had deteriorated, for Méiní distinctly heard them refer to her as a greenhorn. Indeed they may not even have bothered to speak softly for they probably reckoned without Méiní's good knowledge of English. Had she not learned her prayers in that language and been beaten by old Méireas and her mother Máire into speaking it? The word they used was new to her but sensing that it was no compliment, she remembered it for the rest of her life.

She had much to learn, however confident the sight of her aunt had made her. As they walked down the street they passed by a building whose door stood wide open. She peeped in and immediately cowered back to her aunt and the two Ó Criomhthains. 'Christ, Seán!' she exclaimed, 'are they being killed?' The men she had seen lying back in the chairs, the barbers standing over them with razors at the ready, had seemed at first to confirm all the horror tales she had picked up at home about life in America.

Possibly because work was hard to find in Chicopee, or because accommodation was cramped, Méiní soon moved down to Hartford to live with another sister of her father, Kate. She was married to a Corkaguiny man, a Sayers, and she had one son and a daughter, all that remained of four sets of twins of whom the others had failed to survive childhood. Indeed the surviving daughter was herself to die in childbirth some years later.

The Hartford home was comfortable, with five rooms, and must have appeared palatial to Méiní in contrast to the little house at Ballykeen. There were attics in the house, in one of them lived a married couple who were friends and in another a family of French Canadians who had nothing whatever to do with the Irish family down below. The house was a little bit out from the town but close enough to make strolling around the streets – *ag buachailling* as she described it – a favourite occupation of Méiní's leisure time. Soon she had a certain amount of pocket money, for she got a job in a cotton-factory operating a threadmaking machine.

Work ended at one o'clock on Saturdays, and that evening the young people would get together for a dance. They had a special dancehall which was a focus for the young Irish emigrants. If we can judge from her later years, Méiní was always full of divilment, but in one respect she avoided the fashion. While the other girls put paint and powder liberally on themselves, she claimed that in her case the skin that God gave her the first day needed no adornment. She got together a few dollars and bought herself a long dress – like fancy-dress – and of course a hat on her head to turn her very quickly into a real young lady.

All this gallivanting caused her aunt Kate some anxiety. What would she tell them back in Dunquin if any harm should befall their Méiní owing to lack of care by her? Dances started at eight and the aunt made sure she was back at the stroke of twelve. One of the Irish lads would always escort her home. She was friendly with a Blasket girl, Bridie O'Sullivan. Bridie introduced her to some 'Polanders' but Méiní did not hit it off with them as they teased her with comments like 'Irish no good' and 'You've the head of a fool!'

41

Sunday would start early with a trip to Mass followed by a stroll in the country. On Monday, Méiní was up well before six for the start of another gruelling week. By seven o'clock, summer or winter, she was at her workbench and worked through until six in the evening with a break of an hour to have something to eat. On Saturday, work ended at lunchtime after six hours, making a fifty-six hour week in all. Méiní didn't like the work and must have thought ruefully of her complaints about her hard work back at home. As well as this, watching the thread put a great strain on her eyes and she suffered from incessant headaches as a result. For this, Méiní received the equivalent of four shillings a day, which would not have been far short of a week's pay for a servant girl at home.

Romance wasn't long in coming her way; she became friendly with Jimmy Hickey from the Glens near Dingle who had emigrated at about the same time as herself. She would not admit to anything like infatuation, far from it: 'I was and I wasn't in love with him. One foot in and one foot out.' They met every day going and coming in the train which took Méiní to the mill. Back at home they had never met – now in a far land they did their courting in Irish and English as the mood took them. Perhaps the enthusiasm was more on Jimmy's side than Méiní's. He never forgot her and they were to meet again back in Ireland because of enquiries he had made.

The work in the mill was suiting her less and less, and in spite of the attentions of the faithful Jimmy the loneliness for home did not diminish. Aunt Kate was as good to her as any mother, but soon she began to pile up the dollars and cents needed to make the passage home. In this frame of mind she was struck down by a fever. For three weeks she was gravely ill and Dr Lynch, himself an emigrant from Cork, almost despaired of her life. On the third night the crisis was reached and somehow she managed to pull through. For a fortnight she could hardly tell whether she was dead or alive. No tea or milk or coffee were allowed her all that time and once she began to regain her strength, Dr Lynch produced a revolting tonic and warned her to swallow the fill of an eggstand before every meal. If she did this, he promised, she would be better before the bottle was finished. Indeed, within a month, she was back at the mill again. Soon the headaches returned and, seeing this, Aunt Kate came round to agreeing with Méiní that she had better think of going back home. In truth she was afraid that another illness might carry Méiní off and that Máire might say that Kate had neglected her. Just over three years after she had first arrived her passage to Queenstown was booked and she was to leave the land of her birth, this time for ever. There were tears in her eyes as she left her aunt and her two cousins who had become like her brother and sister in those years.

This time she could do the whole journey to the docks by train, and as she travelled from Hartford to New York she must have wondered whether what she was doing was sensible. So many leaving Corkaguiny, and now here she was, travelling against the tide. She had no doubt that she would get a great welcome home – old Méireas was now seventy and was to live another twenty years into the Great War – but it might well be that, back in the cramped little house with no money to fall back on, her four shillings a day she could earn in America would be sadly missed. But no more than in her old age was Méiní one to brood, and if such considerations crossed her mind they would have been quickly dismissed. Was she not a fine girl and were there not fine men in Dunquin who would be glad of a cheerful, hard-working wife? She was nineteen now and it was about time for her to be thinking in those terms.

At the dockside the *Majestic*, the ship that had brought her out, awaited her. Its master was E. J. Smith, afterwards captain of the ill-fated *Titanic*. This time round she had nothing to fear but sea-sickness. She would not have wasted much time looking back at the receding coastline, but after five days, when the word went round that the Fastnet light was again reaching out to them, she rushed to see it. A few more hours and in the dawn light the *Majestic* rounded Daunt's Rock and made for its anchorage outside Cork Harbour. The tender came out to deliver a new batch of emigrants and to collect the few who were now to land at Queenstown. It was but a few steps to the train through the customs shed.

Méiní would soon again be surrounded by people whose home language was Irish and in Dingle itself there would have been many people from her own place. Her first call would have been to Seán O'Shea's pub, which the Dunquin and Ballyferriter men were accustomed to use as their base. Most likely she left her bundle here for collection later and set off on foot through Ventry up over the Clasach. At the highest point of the mountain pass she would have seen at last the Blaskets laid out before her, Inishtooskert, in Seán Ó Riordáin's words, like a statue of a soldier lying on the sea, and beyond it the jagged, inhospitable Tearaght. Coming down through Gleann Luic she could see over to where the little stream, running down the Glen beside the church in Dunquin reached the sea at Béal Átha. Another half-hour and she was home, to the delight of her grandparents and her mother Máire. In no time they were joined by her sister Junie and one or two of her children and soon those of her schoolfriends who still remained in the parish would be calling to inspect the finery she had brought back from the States. Travelling was over except for occasional trips to Dingle and, in her old age, one car-trip to Ballydavid to visit places she had been hearing about all her life. Now she was on the threshold of another adventure, a change by no means expected.

5

NO ROAD WHERE I'M GOING

Once the excitement of her return had died down, both Méiní and her mother began to consider their position. Méiní herself, the wanderlust out of her system, was looking for a suitable husband. Kate Moriarty was delighted to have her back again, and the bond was the stronger because they were both thinking in terms of marriage. Kate had been friendly for some years now with Tomás Phaidí Rua Guiheen, known as 'Plate' and brother to the equally firmly-nicknamed 'Line'. Kate and 'Plate' were eventually to marry in 1901, and when they did Tomás moved from the Blaskets into the Moriarty house in Ballykeen. This fact seems to suggest that he was not well off and this in turn may account for the long courtship.

Tomás's best friend was Seán Eoghain Dunlevy, a widower who lived with his mother and two sons, Eoghan and Maurice, aged twelve and six at that period. Their home was near Castle Point above the Blasket harbour, near the little island graveyard where children were sometimes buried. Seán Eoghain was in his middle thirties, and he got to know Méiní when making up a foursome with 'Plate' and Kate. He was a fine figure of a man, a good singer with a taste for poetry. His rangy presence and tempestuous outgoing personality was calculated to appeal to the girl of spirit that Méiní was. At this stage there seems to have been little to the relationship but a certain flirtatiousness, but Méiní and Kate used to fantasise together about living on the island.

Where the choice of a husband was concerned, Méiní's wishes would have been given some weight, but she would have considered it natural that her mother Máire would expect and demand the final say. When Méiní had been at home for a year or so, Máire decided that she would begin some enquiries, and she approached Seán de Mórdha who lived in Baile an Ghleanna a few fields away, near Paddy Frawley's bridge. Seán was willing to marry her – was she not a fine girl and a knowledgeable and willing worker? – and he agreed to do so provided that she would wait a couple of weeks until he had sold his pigs and put together a few pounds for the marriage expenses. Seán's delaying tactics may have been designed to wheedle a bit extra by way of a dowry out of Máire but, if so, they backfired. Máire was prepared to wait and she came home to report the success of her mission and the fortnight's delay. 'Why so a fortnight?' queried Méiní, her hackles rising. 'Oh he's waiting until he has sold his pigs,' said her mother, 'and then you can go before the priest in Ballyferriter.'

'The curse of the Dún on him!' retorted Méiní. 'If he's that poor I won't marry him. *Ambaist*, I won't get married at all unless you let me have the man I'm inclined to take.'

'And who may that be in God's name?' enquired the anxious mother.

'John Moriarty from Ballykeen and none other.'

'God blast you, that's a man that won't come into this house at any rate!' was the determined reply. Why poor John, Kate's brother, was out of favour we do not know – indeed Méiní may have known that he would not find favour with her mother and was playing for time. The discussion ended with Méiní's enigmatic threat, 'Well, if John doesn't come in I'll make my own match with the man I really want to marry.' Still more enigmatically she added, 'There's no road where I'll be going.'

The next day she told Kate about what had happened and that she was now sure that she would be living on the island. 'Don't count your chickens before they're hatched!' retorted Kate, knowing that Máire would never allow Méiní to marry into the island. Méiní and Kate had many times watched the cruelty of the islanders as they trussed up their animals for transport across the Blasket Sound in their *naomhóga* and some mainland people said that the islanders would be equally cruel to strangers.

Some days later, out from the island with a cow, Seán Eoghain met Méiní as she was walking with Kate on the cliff-top. Sensing that he wanted to be alone with Méiní, Kate moved away. What happened next is best described in Méiní's own words:

'I'm going to ask you as my wife from your mother.'

A blush came to my cheek, the words he spoke gave me such a shock. I thought such a thing would never happen. I admit it was the sweetest sound my ears had ever heard.

'On my soul, my bright love, stay away from her!'

I don't know how I said it, I was so shaken. But when I looked up at the dignified face that was before me, I recognised that he was in earnest. I ran into his arms and kissed him and he kissed me. Kate had gone a little bit away and she didn't bother with what was going on. When my sudden attack of delight had cooled down, I said, 'Stay away from her or the refusal you'll get from her will be the side of the straw-rope. She has a place decided for me but it's not on the island. But I'd prefer you and our patch of the island to the Great State of Russia itself.' So I promised to

47

come the next Saturday and I would be married to him. We made the arrangements together, and then he left me and my pal, and on my soul we had plenty to think about.

Now that the die was cast, the two friends began to count the cost. It was goodbye to Dunquin, goodbye to visiting the Connors in Ballinaraha and their lovely daughters. No more strolling for Méiní to the top of Eagle Mountain or gathering turf with her pals and bringing it home with the ass. From now on they would be far apart with the sea as their boundary ditch. Her youth was gone; she would be a housewife. Her friend's thoughts were equally sad: 'Oh, Méiní,' said Kate, 'the world is a queer strange place. I thought that nothing would ever come between us to drive us away from each other. But I am sad when I think that this may be the last walk we'll take together as young people. The next time we take a walk you'll be a married woman on the island just as you said you'd be. I'm sad to think that we'll be torn apart but that's the way of the world.'

'That's the way it is,' said Méiní, 'but it's the will of God and we have no business to be finding fault with it. We must go through with it but my blessings go with the happy days of my childhood.'

The next Friday evening Seán Eoghain and 'Plate' came in from the Blaskets and they met Méiní just below her sister's house, near the Cuaisín at the Mill River.

'I'll be before you in Ballyferriter tomorrow morning without fail,' said Seán before moving off with 'Plate' on his way to Dingle to make the arrangements. Méiní had her arrangements too. She told her mother that she had been given a message that there was a letter for them to be collected in Ballyferriter and that she and Kate would go in for it early the next day. Suspecting nothing, Máire gave her permission and Méiní arranged to sleep at Kate's house as she often did. Kate had agreed to stand with Méiní as her bridesmaid. The fact that 'Plate' was going to be best man whetted her enthusiasm for the task.

'What a wonderful thing love is!' reflected Méiní in her old age. 'What can it not do? There's nothing else in this world would have got Kate and me out of our sleep in the dark of the morning to go through the showers of snow on the lonely road to Ballyferriter. Nothing but love alone. There wasn't any other thing on the back of the great world that would do it but love took every bit of the poison out of the hardship of the road that was before us.'

Kate and Méiní stayed in Ballyferriter only long enough to pick up a cup of tea when Seán Eoghain arrived with Eoghan de Brún. Eoghan's wife, a daughter of the Blasket poet Seán Dunlevy, was related to Seán Eoghain and their home was in Baile Bhiocáire near Dunquin school. They had just come in from Dingle on Eoghan's mule-cart on which they had gone there the evening before. Early as was the girls' departure from Dunquin, Seán Eoghain and his friends must have left Dingle earlier still. The day was Saturday 25 April 1896 and at nine o'clock Fr John O'Leary, the parish priest, married Seán Eoghain and Méiní. The witnesses were 'Plate' and John Scanlon from Dingle whom they had brought with them that morning.

Once they were safely man and wife, Seán Eoghain, Méiní and their little retinue hurried back to Dingle as fast as their legs and Eoghan de Brún's mule would carry them. While it was unlikely that the news of the wedding would as yet have reached Máire in Dunquin, they thought it better to set off east without delay. In fact it was at eleven o'clock that morning that some local men returning from Ballyferriter brought to Máire the news that Méiní had been married two hours before. The distracted mother made neither stop nor stay until she reached the church at Ballyferriter. Breathless, she went up to the first man she

49

met, as he stood outside a nearby pub:

'Was there any wedding here today that you know of?'

'Indeed there was, ma'am. Seán Dunlevy from the island and your very own daughter.'

'Then 'tis true what I hear tell, and that fellow never asked to marry her!'

In Dingle the wedding-feast was getting under way, the first port of call being Ashe's pub at the head of the quay. The drinks were flowing and the pipes circulating; the friends who had gathered at the news quickly got into party mood. As she sat there, Méiní felt a sense of exhilaration. Wasn't she wed to the man she really wanted, her 'strong, hard and hearty man with his songs and poetry', as she was later to describe him?

The crowd started to disperse as twilight began to set in and the long journey home had to be tackled. But it was not only the road that was on Méiní's mind. She was determined to get to her new island home before her mother would catch her, for Máire would surely wring her neck. In her heart of hearts she knew that the latter's fears were justified; not only was Seán Eoghain a widower and a good fifteen years older than she, but he had two children of his own and his old mother still living in the little island home. In addition, Méiní was a seasoned traveller; the restricted life of the island might be particularly difficult for her to adapt to. Her mother's permission would never have been given to marry Seán Eoghain and Méiní knew that a confrontation would be a distressing experience which must at all costs be avoided.

Eoghan de Brún's mule-cart set out on the road to Dunquin carrying two barrels of porter in order that the wedding could be celebrated on the island also, as would certainly be expected by the neighbours. 'Plate' and Seán Eoghain walked beside the cart; Méiní and Kate rode beside the barrels. It was getting late as they were dropping down through Gleann Luic but nevertheless they were taking no chances. Eoghan de Brún put a blue rug over the two girls in the bottom of the cart just in case Máire was waiting for them along the road.

All was well and they reached Eoghan de Brún's house in Baile Bhiocáire without incident. The mule cart was brought down towards the harbour but the barrels were not left there but at Faill Mhór where the new jetty was built some years later. The Dunquin men would hardly find the porter there; they would assuredly help themselves if they did. The night was spent in drinking, eating and singing in Eoghan de Brún's house; there was always the danger of a sudden arrival in the shape of an enraged Máire. In spite of what must have been their exhaustion after their early start and long foot-slogging of the day before, they decided well before dawn that it was time to go. Méiní left Kate behind her in Eoghan's house; it was a sad goodbye as she set off. As an old woman she recalled her feelings as they parted: 'I followed my own people, for that's what they would now be from that time onwards. I had made an islander out of myself and I'd given the back of my hand to the life of my youth and to the fun and pastimes I had known. 'Twas little I thought that beautiful morning as I left Baile Bhiocáire that all these lovely things would pass away and all my jewels of happiness be taken away from me. But we have to travel these roads if we are to understand the things that must some day come our way.'

Seán Eoghain and Eoghan de Brún made for Faill Chliadh where their *naomhóg* had been tied up the day before. Eoghan had been a great help to Dunlevy, and hospitable to his friends; now he was determined not to miss the celebrations which would take place on the island. Kate may well have persuaded 'Plate' to stay with her on the mainland and Eoghan might have been needed to help Seán Eoghain on the crossing. They brought the *naomhóg* around to Faill

Mhór where Méiní and the barrels were waiting for them, and set out across the Blasket Sound.

It was fully light when they arrived at the Island harbour and at that early hour Peig Sayers was already out, fetching a bucket of water at Pierce Ferriter's well just below Seán Eoghain's house. She watched the *naomhóg* as it approached the harbour below and ran home to report to her husband Patsy 'Flint' who was up early also as a cow was calving: 'Seán Eoghain's down at the harbour and he has Méiní with him.'

'Arrah, what are you saying, woman?' growled Patsy.

'I tell you Seán Eoghain's down at the harbour and a young woman with him. I'm not sure 'tis Méiní but she has all that appearance,' she insisted.

'Well, good luck to him anyway if it is!'

Now that they were safely home, Méiní decided that it was better to lie low, hoping that her mother's wrath would cool down. She knew that Máire would not dare to cross over to the island to confront her in her own home, and she was hopeful that commonsense would eventually gain the upper hand and that she would realise that what could not be cured would have to be endured. The house in Ballykeen was a dull place now that Méiní was gone, and the grandparents were elderly and infirm. Junie, living a short distance away near the mill of Béal Átha, missed her sister and was consumed with curiosity about her life on the island. Blasket people who called on Máire to buy flour would have brought news of Méiní and reported her unwillingness to leave the island for fear of her mother. The first move would have to come from Máire.

Three months after the elopement, Máire sent a message to Méiní by Pats Keane, the island postman and King. She was to come out of the island the following Sunday when the *naomhóga* were coming across for Mass in the Dunquin church at Baile an Teampaill. If the weather was at all suitable, most of the able-bodied men were accustomed to making the crossing, and some of the younger women. The older women did not usually go but would sit together on a stretch of grass near the upper village, facing towards Dunquin and reciting the rosary at the hour of Mass.

Sunday dawned fair and still fearing the tongue-lashing she would get from Máire, Méiní set off with the Massgoers. They reached the old harbour at Dunquin and Méiní began the climb to the cliff-top with growing apprehension. She need not have worried. Back in Ballykeen they had decided to let bygones be bygones, at least as far as Méiní was concerned. A bright welcome awaited her from her mother and sister, and from the old grandparents. Their annoyance at her marriage was forgotten in the joy of reunion: on the table in the weaver's house stood a real treat to welcome her, a bowl of beastings – the first milk from the cow that had calved. The next day when she woke up there was another treat: Máire Keating had placed a goose egg before each of them at the table. A week passed quickly, and before returning with the Blasket people the next Sunday, the whole family went off to Mass together, Máire filled with pride as she showed off her newly-married daughter. When she returned to the island, Méiní brought with her a pet lamb as a wedding present from her mother.

One problem alone remained: Seán Eoghain himself was still not welcome in the house at Ballykeen. After all, he had not asked their blessing before eloping with Méiní, and the runaway marriage had been a blow to their pride. Méiní determined to put matters to rights.

A few Sundays later, the sea in the Blasket Sound was calm enough for another crossing to Mass, and Seán Eoghain and Méiní decked themselves out in their new clothes. There was a light but cold breeze and half-way across Méiní complained to Seán Eoghain that she was feeling cold. He was warm from rowing, so he fell easily into the trap. He handed his new tweed jacket to the shivering Méiní and she kept up the pretence of being cold even when they reached the harbour. Leaving Seán Eoghain with his friends, she set off up the cliff path to visit the Ballykeen family, still with the jacket over her shoulders.

An hour afterwards, Mass was over and the group assembled again at the harbour for the return trip. Méiní arrived late but Seán Eoghain was waiting on the jetty. One thing was lacking: Seán Eoghain's beautiful new jacket: 'God blast you, woman! What have you done with my coat?'

Feigning shock, Méiní lied: 'Isn't it at the cottage above in Ballykeen that I forgot it!'

'Off you go now, girl, and get me back that coat!'

'God blast you, that I will not! You'll go and fetch it your very own self!'

In vain Seán Eoghain cajoled, bullied and swore. In the end, for the other boatmen were getting impatient with their antics, he gave in – that young woman was certainly a vixen! – and up with him to Ballykeen. Pride was swallowed on both sides: he was asked to have a cup of tea, and before he left he had the old couple laughing. Even Máire his mother-in-law was half won over.

On the next trip, Seán Eoghain completed the good work. While Méiní went up to the cottage he made his way to Ballyferriter where he purchased a fine bottle of spirits. Thus armed, he risked a second visit. Soon he and old Seán Keating were sitting at the table matching glass for glass, and Méireas and Máire also had their share. The ice was fully broken.

'Isn't it a fine family we've got for ourselves!' said Seán to his daughter. From then on the maligned Seán Eoghain was a favoured visitor who would bring them fish on his trips to Dunquin, giving old Seán the excuse to get out a bottle and to hear all the latest news from the island.

6

THE ISLAND HOME

In pursuing the peaceful end to Méiní's marriage problems, we have jumped a little ahead of our story and now return to the day of her arrival on the island. As she walked with Seán Eoghain and Eoghan de Brún up the slope from the Nune, as the island harbour was called, past the *stáitsí* on which many *naomhóga* still stood, other islanders apart from Peig and Patsy 'Flint' were beginning their day's work. Passing by some north-facing houses, including the first home of Tomás Ó Criomhthain, the newcomers circled around the *púicín buí*, a storage shed built on the old neolithic corbelling principle. On their right was the lonely island graveyard; here Pierce Ferriter, the renegade poet and warrior, had built his castle where a triangle of land pointed out seawards. Just behind the beehive *púicín* stood Seán Eoghain's south-facing house with its thatched roof.

As they entered, old Máire Boland, Seán Eoghain's mother, rose from her corner to meet the new bride and it was a warm greeting that she gave. At times, Máire was to prove herself cantankerous, but on the whole Méiní was lucky in her mother-in-law. Seán Eoghain's two sons by his previous marriage to 'Lís Criomhthain of Coumeenole, Eoghan who was twelve years of age and Maurice who was six, were still in bed, and we may surmise that their welcome was compounded in equal measure of puzzlement, suspicion and curiosity. What changes could they expect under the régime of this slip of a girl, barely out of her teens? Méiní was always to remain very reticent about these two stepsons; in recounting her life to Mike Pheig Sayers in her old age she mentions them only in the most perfunctory way, and never refers to their childhood. This may reflect tensions, though she certainly remained on friendly terms with Eoghan until the time of her death.

Soon the islanders were gathering around to see the happy pair and to drink their health. Willing hands brought the two barrels of porter from the Nune and there was whiskey and pipes of tobacco galore for the assembled company crowding into the little cottage or sitting outside it in the spring air. Seán Eoghain was, in Méiní's phrase, 'not the man to do them wrong', and the drink flowed as long as the barrels contained a drop.

Sixty years after Méiní's marriage, her nephew Martin Keane gave an account of marriage-night customs in the Blaskets-Dunquin area which may possibly reflect her own experience. When the couple came to their house at night, the oldest woman present would stand up and welcome them before going into the bedroom to arrange the bed. Then she would come down to the fireside and join the company until midnight. Later, as she put the young woman into bed, she would put under her a spray of the herb known as *luibh a' chiorraithe*, a reputed specific against the evil eye and the curse of 'overlooking' so greatly feared. Thus the couple would be guarded against all harm. When the young man came to bed with his bride the old woman would sometimes sleep in the same room, a practice which was supposed to bring luck and a fruitful marriage. In Méiní's case such a duty would normally have fallen to old Máire Boland, but the young boys Eoghan and Maurice would have been in bed a long time before this stage was reached and probably shared the bedroom with the bridal couple. It is unlikely, under the circumstances, that Máire would have considered it necessary to carry out the final part of her duties.

Méiní was up very early the next morning, to begin her day's work by going for a bucket of water at Pierce Ferriter's well. Otherwise known as the Glen Well, this was just seaward of the house at the bottom of a cleft in the ground which formed a boundary of Castle Point, on which the graveyard stood. In years to come it was to be known as Méiní's well. Her natural sense of loneliness must have been all the stronger because of her elopement. Her action had created another Blasket Sound between herself and those she loved. Unlike a mainland bride, there was now little chance for her to visit her home except at long intervals, if indeed she would ever be welcome there again. Seán Eoghain would be back and forward along that stretch of water delivering fish and lobster or collecting supplies but rarely would room be found for her. Even attendance at Mass was to be a rarity, perhaps when the time of the Stations would come around or on odd Sundays when the sea was calm.

On this first morning Méiní did not have time to brood. The celebrations of the previous day had affected Seán Eoghain's mood, so a good breakfast must be waiting for him before he set off on his day's work. It was inevitable also that she should be conscious of her mother-in-law's eyes on her every move, judging her actions not only by her own standards but also by comparison with the methods used by 'Lís Criomhthain before her death.

The breakfast table was no sooner cleared than the old ladies of the lower village came to greet her, as there had been little opportunity for womanly chat the night before. The first to come was Cáit Ó Brien, wife to the island weaver, Eoghan Bán Ó Connor. She and her husband were 'in the soup', that is to say, Protestants, and lived in what had formerly been the 'Souper' mission school, though, in Méiní's phrase, their children were to return 'out of darkness into the light'. Cáit had worked for some years for a doctor in Tralee and Eoghan's brother Paid, who lived in Ventry, had arranged the match between them. Mollín, wife to Tomás Ó Criomhthain's uncle Diarmuid Shea, was the next to come along, with one of the many Mary Kearneys on the island. Soon they were joined by Máire Criomhthain, a sister of Tomás, who was married to Micil O'Sullivan, and was destined to be Méiní's closest island confidante.

Later came Nell Mitchell from Ferriter's Quarter in Dunquin, known as Nell Mhicil after her father, an island midwife and wife to Maurice Phaidí Keane; with her came old Léan Criomhthain, an island grandmother. The remains of the whiskey bottle were consumed and the pipe circulated again while Méiní was being fully quizzed about her life in Dunquin. Máire Criomhthain enquired in particular about Méiní's years in the United States where she herself had spent some time after the death of her first husband, Mártan Keane. There were no wedding presents to be displayed, for her elopement meant that Méiní arrived in the island almost empty-handed. Later on, there was to be the pet lamb and a beautiful bedspread sent to her from the United States by her aunt Mags, who was in her middle thirties at the time of Méiní's marriage. This aunt had helped her mother Máire to rear Méiní during her first two years before Máire's return to Ireland.

7

—

MARRIED LIFE

So began Méiní's life with Seán Eoghain and it was never to be a boring one, for Seán Eoghain was larger than life. His many nicknames – among which were 'Heenan', after a prize-fighter, 'Long John' and 'John the Joker' – indicate that he was a man who made a strong impression on his neighbours. His voice was powerful, so forceful indeed that Robin Flower likened its trumpet-roar of sound to the battle-horn of the Fianna warriors of Irish legend. Tomás Ó Criomhthain says that when Pats Mhicí Keane and Seán Eoghain were arguing together one could hear them three miles from home. Yet his was the voice that could recite poetry with a gentleness that won Méiní's heart, or sing the old traditional songs. He was of an argumentative cast of mind, and as we shall see later he could be contemptuous and dismissive, as on the occasion when he was called on to give his judgement on *An tOileánach* (The Islandman). Physically, he was a man of great height and bodily strength, as the surviving photographs testify, with a large nose and one drooping eye. His strength was combined with a quick temper, and this quality showed itself in the roars and shouts which were inseparable from his dealings with his succession of donkeys.

Allowing for a due meed of wifely exaggeration, Méiní was probably right in claiming that Seán Eoghain was respected by the islanders for being a fine hunter and fisherman. He was certainly great company, the sort of man who gathers an admiring crowd around him when in full flight. He had a tendency to drink too much when he had the opportunity, and Méiní was known to tease him for not being able to hold it. A day at the races in Ventry or in Dingle was entirely to his taste, and he would set off with his friends Mícheál Mhuiris Keane (Nell Mhicil's son) and Patsy 'Flint', Peig Sayers's husband. His gentle side showed itself in his generosity to the many pedlars who so often visited the island to offer their wares, though his lack of English made it difficult to communicate with most of them. In later years at the time of the death of Peig's son he showed great kindness to the stricken mother and ailing father in their loneliness and despair.

As a widower, Seán Eoghain claimed to know everything that was to be known about the fair sex: Tomás had on one occasion to back him up in an argument with four girls about female beauty. By no means did he put his new bride on a pedestal and he was not beyond personal remarks at her expense. During a storm he claimed that he had seen the sea turn red. When Méiní asked sceptically what had made it red that day, he retorted, 'The same God who turned your skin yellow!'

For all his loud bluster, the young Méiní knew how to keep him under control. She knew, for example, that he was a slave to many superstitions which she did not share, and as the story of the cat will later show, he had in full measure that fear of the unknown which had been passed on from the spiritual frame of his ancestors. Theirs was to be a marriage of equals, his larger than life qualities fully balanced by Méiní's lively, gentle mocking humour and feminine wiles, a relationship of reciprocal regard and interaction which grew closer as the passing years made the initial gap in their ages – for he was fully fifteen years older than Méiní – seem less and less of consequence.

Although in the first days of her marriage Méiní bore a deep sense of guilt because in marrying Seán Eoghain she had defied her mother, the home in which she found herself was a busy one and there was little time to brood. Máire Boland liked to keep control of the household, and in addition felt a particular sense of responsibility for Méiní's stepsons. This left Méiní free to accompany her husband and to help him with much of his work. On wet days and in the dark evenings there was no lack of company. Not only did Máire have her own friends but also those who had been friends of 'Lís Criomhthain, the first wife. Among those who visited old Máire was a group who gave Méiní an insight into what life was like on the island back into the early years of the nineteenth century. First came old Mící Keane, known as 'Mící Barr a' Bhaile' as he lived in the upper village. He was by now badly crippled, but made at least one trip each day to visit his daughter Máire who was married to Tomás Ó Criomhthain. Before returning he would visit Máire Boland and pass on the news of the day to Seán Eoghain. Mící was the father of the island king Pats Mhicí Keane who as island postman was the main source of news, since he collected the post from Dunquin twice a week. The news his son brought would be passed on by Mící to his friends. When stop press items were in short supply, Máire and Mící never tired of mulling over the hardships of their early life, savouring in particular memories of their struggles with the landlord's agents.

Another regular visitor was Mícheál Guiheen, known as 'Flint', now in his late sixties, and Peig Sayers's father-in-law. They would be joined frequently by Paidí Rua Guiheen, father of 'Line' Guiheen and of Tomás – or 'Plate' – whom we have already met as Seán Eoghain's best man.

Just across the way stood the Islandman's original home, but even though he had moved into his new house behind Seán Eoghain's there was still plenty of coming and going between the two families. Seán Dunlevy, the island poet, was in the last years of his life, and his visits to his cousin Seán Eoghain were rare events – his son-in-law Eoghan de Brún had provided transport for the elopement.

Beside Seán Eoghain's house was that of Eileen, widow of Tomás 'Maol' Kearney (the epithet preventing confusion with the man of the same name who was the father of Pats Tom of whom we shall hear more). Eileen was 'the old hag across the way' of whom Ó Criomhthain wrote so scathingly. Her son Pat (Paid Thomáis) was an eccentric individual of uncertain but belligerent temperament, described by Méiní as a puny scatterbrained little man. He made free of Seán Eoghain's household and regaled Máire and Méiní with his stories. His favourite was that of the *Rolling Swan*, a sailing-ship which went aground on the north of the island at Cuas Fhaill Beag during his boyhood. The crew were saved when a local woman named Mary Doody volunteered to pilot the ship to safety as the tide lifted her free. Pat's fondness for telling tales of his boyhood was equalled only by his liking for tittle-tattle about his neighbours and he seems to have been an unpopular and lonely figure.

When these old friends of hers were not there to spark her into reminiscence, Máire Boland took great delight in telling Méiní her stories of her youth and married days, and some of these Méiní has passed on. She and her husband had suffered grievously at the hands of landlords and their agents, and her accounts gain authenticity from her mention of the occasional acts of kindness which they performed. Bess Rice of Fahan, whose name is prominent among those earmarked as tyrants in the island story, attracted special loathing. Méiní asked Máire why she never said the conventional phrase of blessing on the dead when she talked about Bess and her workers. 'God would not allow me,' was her answer. 'If I were to tell you what they did you would not believe it.' Máire and her long-dead husband Johnnie Dunlevy had the roof taken off their house for arrears of rent even though they were pitifully poor. When wrongfully accused of non-payment, Máire had gone herself to interview Bess in her home and the matter was eventually adjusted. On another occasion their sheep were driven off the hillside and sold on the mainland. 'Oh, Méiní,' Máire used to say, 'ours was a dark, dark world.'

Mention has already been made of one other older woman, Máire Criomhthain, sister of the Islandman. Her second husband, Micil O'Sullivan was brother to Eoghan O'Sullivan, the 'Daideo' of *Twenty Years A-Growing*, Maurice O'Sullivan's grandfather. Micil and Máire had at least five children born between 1873 and 1884, and their first child Seán Mhicil remained on the island and brought up a musical family. Their daughter 'Lís married on the island a son of Seán Mhicíl Kearney, Seán, known as 'Seásaí'. Even though Máire was a whole generation older than Méiní, having been married for the second time in 1872, they had a strong attachment to one another, and Méiní was allowed into the circle of her friends who met around her spinning-wheel. Since as a widow Máire had spent some years in America, they had much to talk about, and much of the time, when alone, they spoke in English. To her Méiní gave credit for the survival of her own command of English, but, even more important, she said it was from Máire that she gleaned many of the stories which in her old age were collected from her. Máire was quite clearly a woman of spirit and a natural leader; Méiní's strong spirit and downright, humorous yet compassionate personality would understandably attract her. She was by far the closest friend of the young Méiní in her first years on the island and took the place of the mother and grandmother now divided from her by the treacherous waters of the Blasket Sound.

For some years her mother-in-law was still strong enough to do most of the work around the little house, indeed she insisted on doing so, and so Méiní had plenty of time for visiting. Not that the domestic work was very exacting at the best of times – the furnishings of the house were traditional and very basic. A wooden dresser, a rough deal table, a few niches in the wall to act as cupboards, and one or two rope-seated *súgán* chairs by the fireside. About the only food that had to be bought was flour or Indian meal to make the 'cake' over the fire, and sugar and tea in small quantities. Everything else could be had on the island and prepared by the families themselves. Salted pork and fish kept in barrels got them over the winter days. In the warmer days there was fish in plenty, though lobsters were rarely if ever eaten by the fishermen who caught them. Mrs Thompson, in her *Brief Account of the Change in Religious Opinion . . . in Dingle and the West of Kerry* (1846), tells how the island women kept a supply of seaweed in their pockets which they chewed incessantly. This was 'dulse' or *dileasc* and would still have been dried and chewed in Méiní's young married life. A hot dish called 'sladdy' was also made in which a certain type of seaweed, sea-lettuce or sea-laver, was boiled and stirred for hours and eaten as a thick soup. This was classed along with butter, meat and fish as *anlann* or 'kitchen', which term covered tasty food used to supplement the basic diet of potatoes, bread and milk. Sea-grass was traditionally collected on Good Friday.

Sea-gulls' eggs were a delicacy, as collecting them was a hazardous occupation. When one of his sons brought some of them home, Seán Eoghain, according to Tomás Ó Criomhthain, praised them, saying that such poultry cost nothing to keep, 'a far cry from the useless collection of hens in the house that gobble half a bag of meal every month'.

The women of the house baked the bread each day, and

Tomás tells how Seán Eoghain put a newly-baked loaf on the windowsill outside the house to cool it down, only to suffer the humiliation of having it stolen. On another occasion a field of his turnips was raided and he blamed the men who were going down to the *naomhóga* at night.

At the time of Méiní's marriage, conditions in some of the Blasket houses were very poor. Not until 1907 when the Congested Districts Board took over the islands and granted tenancies to the islanders did conditions begin to improve. Some of the worst houses were near Castle or Ferriter's Point, immediately facing Seán Eoghain's house. After his marriage Tomás Ó Criomhthain left one of these and built himself a new house a few yards to the north, facing south like the other houses. In 1910 the position was further relieved by the building of five new mainland-facing two-storey houses high up at Slinneán Bán, into one of which Peig Sayers and her family moved. Where Méiní was concerned, she was married for nearly a quarter of a century before anything was done by Seán Eoghain to increase the accommodation in her little house.

8

FIRING AND FISHING

As soon as Seán Eoghain announced to his bride of a few months that the turf was ready to be brought back home, Méiní set off with her mother-in-law for her first journey to the hill. Trips in search of turf, leading a donkey with its panniers hanging at each side, were not of course a novelty to Méiní: she had made many trips up the Clasach road on similar errands for her mother and grandfather. In the Blaskets such trips were to occupy a large part of her working life for many years. Seán Eoghain's turf bank was at Mullach Reamhar, on the second-highest hill on the island, near to where the soldiers who operated the signal-tower had cut their turf in the old days. The view was breathtaking and on her first visit Méiní was scared of the precipitous slopes on either side which she had not been used to back at home. She records that as she looked across at Dunquin and pointed out her home to old Máire, she felt even more strongly the doubts which she had felt on her first arrival. In spite of this, it was not long before she was laughing heartily at the rabbits dancing on the hill. Her mother-in-law teased her about the Dunquin people and Méiní stood up for them, but she did not strengthen her case when Máire noticed how scared she was that the donkey would fall into the sea.

What timid creatures these mainlanders were!

On her second trip she was more confident, for it was with Seán Eoghain that she went up by the Top of the Two Glens. Her husband was convinced that some of his neighbours would steal his turf unless he kept a very close eye on it, and for this reason he himself made regular trips to check up. This was all the more necessary since the turf on the island was beginning to run out. Méiní was glad of his company on her first few runs as, not only was she scared of the slopes, but she was also terrified in case the donkey might tumble into the sea or down the cliff-edge.

Tomás Ó Criomhthain cut turf in the same bog as Seán Eoghain up by the old tower, and many a story was swapped as they met on the slope to the bog or when resting from their back-breaking work. The Islandman found Seán Eoghain extremely good company and wrote copiously about him in *Allagar na hInise* (Island Cross-Talk), especially about his infamous donkeys. One fine day he went to find the ass to draw some turf and spent most of the day in a fruitless search north and west. Meanwhile, at home, Méiní was given the news that the donkey was stuck on a cliff-ledge on the south of the island. By this time she had overcome her fear of heights and she decided to scramble down to rescue the donkey. The result was that neither she nor the donkey could go up or down, and their rescue had to await the arrival of Seán Eoghain and some of his friends with a long stout rope.

Méiní was involved on another occasion when Seán Eoghain, bawling loudly as was his wont, drove the current donkey down the hill towards home only to start a cavalry charge among the houses of the lower village. Méiní heard the commotion and rushed out with arms outstretched to head him off. Such however was the slope of the hill that the donkey sailed over her head with one bound, and, turning tail, set off up the hill again.

Seán Eoghain enjoyed so much passing the time of day with the neighbours whom he met on the road to the bog that the ass frequently wandered off. In his later years he had a habit of dozing off in the chair while Tomás read to him and on one of these occasions his errant donkey fell down the cliff at Seals' Cove. On a later occasion a new ass he had bought in Ventry for thirty shillings disgraced him by tearing a neighbour's bag of flour and then wandering off on to the White Strand. The impression persists that Seán Eoghain was an inconsiderate master, combining neglect with fierce bursts of temper. Tears of laughter streaming down his cheeks, Robin Flower told Kruger Kavanagh one day how Seán Eoghain in a tantrum had thrown his latest donkey over a 150-foot cliff. Although the story is otherwise unauthenticated, it accords very well with Seán Eoghain's fiery temperament.

A photograph survives showing Méiní in middle age returning from the bog with her dog and a fully loaded donkey, but this was far from being her only outside work. Wearing her red skirt, she would feed the hens of which Seán Eoghain so disapproved; there were also potatoes to be earthed up and saved and the newly-cut oats to be tied up. The more of this work that Méiní could do, the more time was left free for Seán Eoghain to go fishing and hunting rabbits, seals, and seabirds or their eggs. Méiní was particularly proud of her husband's skill as a hunter, which often took him far afield to the other islands, particularly to Inishvickillane and to the Tearaght for puffins. He told old Eoghan O'Sullivan that in his opinion God had put the seals in the sea so that poor people would have plenty to eat even though they hadn't got the price of a pig. Although the seal oil was valuable for the little *sligí* or cresset-lights which served before the use of paraffin-lamps became widespread, there was a certain stigma attached to eating their flesh and the custom all but died out during Seán Eoghain's lifetime.

Mike Pheig has recounted how Méiní used to dread the beginning of the fishing season because Seán Eoghain left her bed and took off with the rest of his crew, often spending a whole week away from home. Her heart would be in her throat as the mackerel season started. 'Make the tea, Méiní,' Seán Eoghain would say, 'for I must be on my way out now. There's every appearance of mackerel in the Blasket road tonight.'

After 1890 there were no big boats on the island; prior to that the upper and lower villages had a good solid fishing-boat apiece. In that year the boats were seized by the bailiffs for non-payment of rent and rotted away unbid for on the quayside in Dingle. The islanders had no option but to adopt the *naomhóg* or tarred-canvas currach which had been originally introduced into the area by the Hartneys of County Clare. These boats were easily replaceable and not worth the landlord's trouble to confiscate. They demanded particular skill in managing them but they were adaptable and seaworthy craft. Inevitably they were looked on as less safe than the larger boats had been, especially by wives and sweethearts, and Méiní was not free of that dread.

Sometimes the journeys were quite far afield; the Blasket fishermen would visit the little Skellig in search of the young of the gannet. Tomás records a belief that gannets would stand on no dry land except on marble, and the reddish marble on this island had a large population. When visiting Iveragh the islanders would call at places like Portmagee. Maurice Mhuiris Keane tells of a visit there with Seán Eoghain in the early days of his marriage to Méiní. When ashore, the islanders were not averse from a bit of fun, and Seán Eoghain was as fond as the next man of a drinking session when the opportunity offered. On this occasion the islanders called in at Inishvickillane on the return journey and were treated with characteristic hospitality by 'old Maurice Daly' and his wife Cáit Guiheen.

During the season it was around the latter island that Seán Eoghain and his crew most often did their fishing. It was quite normal for them to be away from Monday to Saturday and during this time there was no contact with home to offset the anxieties of their womenfolk. In their small craft it was essential for their safety that they should be able to read the signs and the seasons. Bursting in on his friend Tomás with talk of bad weather in prospect, Seán Eoghain tells of disturbances in the balance of nature – otters living on shore, seals walking the land, and, another very bad sign, Beiginis white with seagulls. And it was not only the weather that was lying in wait for them. When the captain of the lobster-boat refused to buy their lobsters Seán Eoghain knew exactly why: 'Isn't that fellow a Corkman and haven't you heard for long enough that they're the worst crowd in Ireland? May Satan sweep that fellow away!' On another occasion the carters at Dunquin were on strike because the buyers had reduced their payments and the fishermen couldn't get their fish to market. Or again, the French fishing-boats had put down lobster-pots among the islanders' own pots and not a penny of the proceeds went to local men. Seán Eoghain was not by temperament inclined to accept trouble in a philosophic spirit: one can imagine him ranting and raving, surrounded by his friends who are stirring him up to ever greater feats of eloquence and invective.

When Máire Boland eventually became too old to look after the household, in the years preceding her death, the centre of gravity of Méiní's life moved away from the turf-bog and the fields. Apart from the routine daily chores, she spent many hours knitting socks and *geantsaís* for her menfolk; this in turn involved combing, drawing, dyeing and spinning her own wool from the island sheep. Various traditional dyes had been used in earlier times, and in fact the earliest chests of tea that floated ashore from wrecks were chiefly valued for the dye the tea provided. In Méiní's day commercial dyes were coming into use, though much of the wool was left in its natural colour.

Méiní gives an interesting picture of work parties among the island women at the home of Máire Criomhthain. The latter was clearly a strong-willed woman, and while she was spinning other island women would be sitting around her and not one of them but would be carding wool or knitting or sewing. Sometimes Máire and Méiní would break into English as they almost invariably did when they were alone. 'Many times the other women used to say we were like the Greeks.' The Dingle people at that time used to make fun of the islanders' bad English; in her old age, Méiní recorded with pride that 'the respect then held for English is now held for our native language.'

As Méiní sat listening to Máire telling her stories, she used to close her eyes and imagine that she was back in her grandmother's house above Faill Chliadh, sitting with her friend Kate as an old beggar-woman told stories literally for her supper. Méireas, she tells us, was rarely without a beggar in the house – there was always a bed for the poor, and those that could tell a good tale or bring news of the wider world were especially welcome.

9

HASTE TO THE WEDDING

About a year after her marriage, Méiní was awaiting her first child. As summer drew to an end, she decided to return to her mother for the birth. When her time was coming near she set off across the Blasket Sound. Her first call in Ballykeen was to Kate Moriarty; she felt guilty because of her elopement and thought that her people might say that she was crawling home only when she needed help. In such a case, she thought that Kate's presence would take the poison out of the story. 'Nowadays,' she said in her old age, 'I could marry a black man and there'd be no shame.' Kate's calming presence proved unnecessary, for 'You'd think I came down from heaven.' On 9 September 1897, a boy was born and Seán Eoghain made his way from the Blaskets as soon as word reached him. The news could not have been better; now he would have a fisherman to help him in his old age, an expectation which was to be amply fulfilled.

The first requisite was to celebrate the birth and that necessitated whiskey. Fortunately, Máire 'Chuainí' who lived a couple of hundred yards away down by Béal Átha ran a rudimentary shebeen. From her, Seán Eoghain purchased two bottles of the best whiskey and old Seán Keating got another bottle. The midwife and Méiní's mother helped the men and the visitors to empty them. Before the baptism on 14 September there was some disagreement as to what the child should be called, but Seán Eoghain insisted that he be called after his brother Séamus who had been born in 1868 and had been killed by a train in America. When the ceremony was over the proud father returned to the island with Méiní and her son. There the real celebrations began, and ten bottles of whiskey – so the story persists – were drunk. Old Máire Boland was filled with delight and took over the management of the child as much as Méiní would allow her. A new teat and milk bottle were brought back from the mainland and one of the many cradles that were unused in the island houses was borrowed.

In the next few years, Méiní was pregnant several times, but no child survived until a girl was born in April 1903. This time, no name was possible but Máire, the name of the child's mother, two grandmothers and great-grandmother. In her old age, Méiní told Mike Pheig Sayers that Máire had been born within a year of Séamus's birth. She may have been thinking of an earlier daughter who did not survive birth and whom she may have thought of as Máire also.

By the time his young sister was born, Séamus was reaching the age when he could be sent to school, and at this stage his step-brother Maurice would still have been a pupil. During his first years at school there were three changes of teacher and this may have meant that Séamus got off to a bad start. Liam Boland, brother of Peig's friend Cáit Jim, left the island school in 1904 and was replaced by Arthur Beckett who stayed for two years. In 1906 Thomas Savage arrived from Lixnaw and he was able to give badly needed stability to the school, remaining as he did for eighteen years. In September 1907 a second teacher, Kate Manning, was sent to the island. She was a local woman who in 1921 married Maurice and became a part of Méiní's household. In spite of Savage's arrival, Séamus did not

improve in his schoolwork and missed many days. Thinking
that if she sent him to Master Ó Dálaigh in Dunquin school
he would be easier to discipline, Méiní arranged for him to
go and live with his grandmother when he was about ten
years of age. This unsuccessful experiment was quickly
abandoned; during his period on the mainland he hardly
spent two days in school. By this stage young Máire was
getting up to school age. She was to have all her schooling
on the Blaskets and was competent in the three Rs when
she left.

One of the main diversions on the island was the excitement
associated with matchmaking and the occasional wedding
that resulted. One wedding, in 1901, so stood out in Méiní's
memory that she retained the impression that it was the
first after her own arrival. This ceremony was probably
unique in that it was a double wedding in which all four
principals were Blasket islanders. The first pair were Maurice
Keane ('Maras Mhuiris') whose stories were published as *Ar
Muir is ar Tír* (*Land and Sea*) in 1991, and Cáit Kearney,
daughter of Seán Mhichíl and Cáit Mitchell (Cáit Shilbhí)
from Ferriter's Quarter in Dunquin. The second pair were
Cáit Kearney's brother Pat ('Filí') and Nell O'Connor,
daughter of Eoghan Bán the island weaver and Cáit O'Brien,
both of whom we have already met.

Maurice Keane has described himself how four *naomhóga*
set out from the Blaskets, two of them carrying his own
wedding party and the other two the party of 'Filí'. The first
job was to get the marriage licences from the priest and
when this was done they stayed in Dingle until the next day.
Two coaches were hired and they set off for Ballyferriter
where Fr O'Leary married them. After the wedding they
went to Muiris de Hora's where a beginning was made on
the celebrations. As it drew towards evening the party made
its way to Dunquin and at Fáill Chliadh they found a fleet

of island *naomhóga* waiting for them. The convoy set out across the Blasket Sound and on their arrival the wedding feast began in earnest, apparently at Eoghan Bán's house, the old Soupers' school. Nine barrels of Bandon Rattler, brewed by Allmans in west Cork, were consumed at this feast, according to Méiní, and the fact that in Maurice Keane's memory it was eight barrels plus a gallon of whiskey confirms that it was certainly an occasion when thirsty souls were amply refreshed. 'Seáinín an Cnagaire' was brought from the mainland to provide fiddle music for the dancers, and no doubt the island musicians did their share.

There was a dramatic interlude: the festivities were interrupted by the arrival of the crazy woman of the island. This was Máire Kearney, the aunt of two of the principals. The terrible condition she was in, hair matted and clothes dishevelled, caused a tremor among the guests who were dressed in their best clothes. Máire's husband had been drowned while fishing from a rock at Inishtooskert and a year afterwards, according to Méiní's account, her little daughter was lost when a high tide carried off her hut from the cliff edge. The distracted mother's mind had given away under this double tragedy and she continued to wander about the island, calling loudly and refusing hospitality from her neighbours. In her first days on the island, Méiní had taken fright when she heard Máire's loud wailing in the darkness. Now at the wedding feast, having been pressed to take some food, she stood in the frame of the door as she was leaving and addressed the assembly in a way which remained vividly in Méiní's mind sixty years later: 'Thanks be to God,' she said, 'that I have eaten this supper at the wedding of my own brother's son, and my own girl floating on the wave leaving me wandering without a roof over my head.' When the distracted old woman went out into the dark, the wedding feast started in earnest. Méiní noticed that Maurice Keane's mother, Nell Mitchell, had a particular fondness for the porter but there was plenty for everyone and 'Seáinín an Cnagaire' played some jigs. Méiní went home with Máire Criomhthain when the women took their departure. Seán Eoghain and his pals had no intention of leaving while any Bandon Rattler still remained.

These were busy times, for only four days before the double wedding Méiní and Seán Eoghain had been to the mainland for the wedding of their close friends, Tomás Guiheen and Kate Moriarty, the best-man and bridesmaid of five years before. Méiní says that this was shortly after Máire's difficult birth, but she must have been referring here again to a child who did not survive as the Máire who lived was not born until two years later. When Kate invited Méiní to come to her wedding, the latter was careful to ask permission of Máire Boland who was still nominal ruler of the household and she undertook to look after the three boys. Cáit O'Brien, whose own daughter was to be married within the week came over to stay with old Máire. She had worked in a doctor's house and was used to managing old people.

Méiní's first visit in Dunquin was to her mother who wept with joy to see her daughter. She had brought her a present of some rabbits which Seán Eoghain had caught in Inishnabro the day before. As Méiní found herself in the middle of a big crowd in Ballyferriter where Patrick Sayers and Cáit Garvey from Ferriter's Quarter were also being married that day, her thoughts returned to the exciting times she and Cáit had shared in their schooldays – raiding birds' nests was their particular delight.

Tomás and Kate settled down in her home in Ballykeen and raised a large family there. Her brother Maurice ('Piley') will be met at a later stage. Before her marriage Kate had spent six months on Inishvickillane in the house of Maurice Daly whose wife Cáit Guiheen was a relation of hers. The stories which Kate brought back from the Inish so interested

Méiní that she hoped to visit the island herself, an ambition not to be fulfilled.

At that time the almost invariable custom in the area was for matches to be made in the days between Christmas and the Epiphany (Little or Women's Christmas). The weddings would then take place before Lent, on a Tuesday or a Saturday, the last possible day being Shrove Tuesday. The majority of local weddings were thus celebrated in February or early March. In Ballyferriter, six weddings might be held in one day, as happened in 1892 when Peig Sayers and Patsy 'Flint' Guiheen were married. Méiní's own wedding after Easter was thus out of line with what would have been expected, at a time when her mother would have suspended her matchmaking enquiries until the following Christmas. In this connection, grandmother Méireas and Máire were reputed to hold the secret of the black saucepan. This was a love potion which, on being given to a man, made him fall in love with a girl. In North Kerry, the reputed ingredient of the *sáspan dubh* is the droppings of a white gander, and a similar love potion has been reported from Turkey. It may have been that Máire looked on this charm as a further weapon in her matchmaking armoury, but all her plans were circumvented by Méiní's elopement.

10
##

DISTINGUISHED VISITORS

At home on the island, especially when there were young visitors to excite the romantic interests of the young islanders, dances were organised. Rory 'Roger' O'Kennedy from Letteragh used to come to the island to teach dancing and stayed in Méiní's house, stretching out on the settle. Every evening he used to play for dancing and he taught many a person to dance well. Although of a resilient temperament, Méiní inevitably suffered from bouts of depression aggravated by the loss at birth of some of her children and from homesickness for her home and friend Kate in Dunquin. On such occasions, nothing cheered her up as much as a visit from Roger and all the excitement associated with the dances which he organised in the houses.

It was customary for a few *naomhóga* to set out for the mainland, if the weather was sufficiently calm, when news came of a dance being organised at the Móinteán on the cliffs at Dunquin or even at the top of the Clasach road to Ventry. *An tOileánach* records an occasion when Maitiú the island fiddler accompanied them and provided the music for the mainland dance. In the 1920s there seems to have been a resurgence of musical talent. Pádraig Keane ('Casht') was a fine musician and was eventually followed as a fiddler by his son Seán. Junie Dunlevy (Junie Mháire Eoghain) was herself a fine singer and a granddaughter of the poet Seán Dunlevy. Her sons Seáinín Sullivan ('Seáinín Mhicil'), Paddy and Mike were violinists and I have heard the latter described as the best musician of them all. Other musicians in these and succeeding years were Paddy O'Connor (Paddy Eoghain Bháin), Tom Daly of the Inish, Mike O'Sullivan (The Tailor – brother of the author Maurice) and the two Kearney cousins Seán 'Filí' and Seán 'Sheásaí'. The latter's sister 'Lís and Peats Guiheen, husband of the storyteller Gobnait Kennedy, were also accomplished musicians. The melodeon became a popular instrument which was played by Seán Tom Kearney, Cáit Sheásaí Kearney, the children of Mícheál Keane (Buffer) and Mag an Rí who was married to the King's son Seán and came from Ballinclea near Ventry. Although not all this range of musicians was available at any one time, or indeed could claim equal talent, the number involved was remarkable in such a small community, even allowing for the long winter evenings when the villagers were housebound with ample time for practice.

Dances were held regularly in the schoolhouse, which, along with the Dáil – the house at the top of the village which belonged to Máire Scanlon and her husband the *Poncán* – and to some extent Peig Sayers's house up in Slinneán Bán, performed some of the functions of a modern community centre. Sunday was a favourite day for holding the island dances. Séamus Kavanagh from Gleann Luic ('Séamus Twoee') used to cross over each summer Sunday in the period of the Great War and the 1920s with a group of lads from Dunquin, to dance in the schoolhouse until ten or eleven o'clock at night. Such meetings partly account for the high rate of intermarriage between islanders and mainland people. Inhabitants of the villages which stretched out between Ventry on the south around by Slea Head and north as far as Brandon mountain quite frequently married into island families and prevented excessive inbreeding, a danger in such a close-knit community.

Every Tuesday and Friday when conditions made it possible, Pats Mhicí Keane, the king of the island, set off in his *naomhóg* to collect the island post from the mainland. Often when returning he would bring back visitors for a stay and they would usually lodge at his own house. An early visitor in Méiní's time was John Millington Synge. He arrived in August 1905 and stayed for some weeks in Pats Mhicí's house, looked after by his elder daughter Máire, who was about twenty at the time. His visit was of importance in providing us with a closely observed description of the island life, and inspired him to poetry. Méiní records how he went around making pencil sketches, and his photographs are among the earliest taken on the island. She expresses surprise that Synge stayed so long there, because the villagers, amused by his strange gait, constantly made fun of him. 'If I had been in his shoes,' Méiní comments, 'I wouldn't have stayed one week on the island. He didn't understand the mockery that the islanders were directing at him and they didn't know that he was writing about them.' The islanders did not dislike Synge but they were deeply hurt when they read his descriptions which became part of *In Wicklow and West Kerry*. One passage which caused them particular offence was clearly meant by Synge as a tribute to their hospitality: he describes how, without asking him whether he were hungry, they started to prepare tea and rashers and bacon. His hostess Máire took this as a criticism of her hospitality, even though Synge in the same passage pays a tribute to her beauty. She may also have considered as somewhat distasteful his reference to her delicate feet and ankles, which he contrasts with those of the other island women. His description of the poor furnishings of the house and the expedients necessary to ensure his comfort were undoubtedly painful to such proud and independent people. It is greatly to be regretted that the Blasket people felt hurt by what Synge had written about them. While he was with them they looked on him as a harmless and amiable eccentric and a butt for private jokes although his writing expresses a warm sensitivity to the culture and society of the island. There is no suggestion of any cheap gibes at the islanders' expense which would have justified the hurt pride to which his written account gave rise.

The islanders may have been unduly sensitive to the poor standard of material comfort which was their lot but, poor as it was, they were prepared to share it. Méiní tells of visits by many beggars to the island, including one old Galway woman whose Irish sounded harsh and jarring. As a general rule, the islanders found the beggars more to their taste than the scholarly visitors, because they were able to earn their keep by telling stories or reciting poems as few of the scholars were willing or able to do. Méiní's mother and grandparents had always given hospitality to beggars in Dunquin, and she herself carried on this tradition in the island. After all, little was needed except some straw in front of the fire and a meal of potatoes and fish.

In 1910 the most faithful of all the island's friends arrived for the first time. This was Robin Flower, affectionately nicknamed *Bláithín* (little flower) who had come at the suggestion of Carl Marstrander, the Scandinavian Celtic scholar who had spent some months in the island, studying with Tomás Ó Criomhthain in 1907. Although Méiní does not tell us anything new about Marstrander, she can hardly have failed to see him as he made his way down from the King's house in the Upper Village for his lessons with Tomás whose house was a few yards behind hers.

Flower's trips to the Blaskets have been much written about, both by himself in *The Western Island* (1944) and by other scholars. His near-yearly visits paid rich dividends in his recording of stories from Peig Sayers and Tomás. This gifted scholar, Keeper of Manuscripts at the British Museum, brought his wife and children to the island after his marriage and they mixed at leisure and in school with the island community. Méiní does not claim to have had a great deal to do with Bláithín on a regular basis, but he clearly knocked a great deal of fun out of Seán Eoghain and in his book describes a visit to Méiní's home. By the time of this visit, Méiní's stepson Maurice was married to an island school-mistress, and Seán Eoghain is shown dandling their daughter on his knee. A warm greeting to his visitor is followed by Seán Eoghain with an instruction to Méiní to wet the tea. When Bláithín turns down the offer, a discussion erupts about the evil effects of tea and sugar, until it is cut short by the arrival of Gobnait Kennedy, a mainlander from the Gorta Dubha who is married to Pats Guiheen, and one of the best storytellers on the island. In response to their pleas she consents to tell the oft-repeated story of Purty Deas Squarey.

Bláithín's sojourns in the King's house ended when the Princess, Cáit, married John Casey of Dunquin in 1918. From then on he stayed with Máire, Cáit's elder sister and his former hostess, who lived in the next house up as the wife of Mike Léan Guiheen. She had been Synge's little hostess in 1905 and was reputed to be the prototype of Pegeen Mike in *The Playboy of the Western World*.

Not all the visitors who had business in the island were scholars. There were visiting tradesmen too. Gobnait's own father, Dan Kennedy, was a stonemason and a weaver who regularly came to the island from his home near Ballyferriter to visit his daughter and to help in building any new houses that were required. When the island weaver, Eoghan Bán O'Connor, became too old to carry on his trade in the Soupers' School, Dan Kennedy would bring over in the summer, when any building took place, the cloth which he had woven during the winter. From Ferriter's Quarter in Dunquin came the tailor Scanlon, father of Máire Scanlon who lived at the very top of the village with her husband Thomas Kearney. He was known as the *Poncán* – or Yank – in tribute to his widebrimmed Western-style hat, though he had never been to the States. Máire we shall meet again as an assistant midwife to Méiní. Her house was known as the *Dáil* because it was a meeting and discussion place for the young of the island and a frequent venue for dances and storytelling. Its proximity to the Yank's well (*Tobar a' Phoncáin*) made it a natural meetingplace. When Scanlon arrived on the island to make whatever garments were required, his custom was to take a cottage door off its hinges and use it as a workbench. He would stay a fortnight making flannel and tweed trousers for the men and boys, and long-sleeved waistcoats for the old people.

Visitors like Kennedy and Scanlon were important in keeping links between their native communities and the island people, and in bringing news of eligible bachelors and potential brides for the young people of the island, as happened in the case of their own daughters. Not that islanders were content to sit back and let the world come to them. Seán Eoghain was always keen for a trip to Dingle or to the races, with the emphasis on some hard drinking, and on such occasions Méiní was only too glad to accompany him. Before 1890 when the upper and lower villages each had their own large boat, big numbers of the island people could make the Christmas expeditions, but by the time of Méiní's marriage the islanders had to rely completely on *naomhóga*. At least one person from each house would set out for Dingle to bring back the groceries and some gallons of stout for the Christmas feasting. Candles were very important for extra lighting and as beacons in the windows from Christmas Eve to Little Christmas. Sometimes if it was possible to get across to Mass on Christmas Day, a party of the younger islanders would remain on the mainland to join the Wren groups on St Stephen's Day. This was a day of intense activity in and around the pubs in Dingle town and money would be made by following the island Wren from village to village. In each house they visited, the island musicians would play a tune or two. Back in the Blaskets things were unnaturally quiet until the young people got back again. Then the Christmas spirit would return and games of football and rudimentary hurling would be played on the White Strand, the more impetuous spirits soaked through as a result of retrieving the ball from the icy water.

On one of her trips to Dingle some years after her marriage, Méiní was hailed in the street by Pats Tom Kearney, calling her to come and meet a returned Yank. It turned out to be none other than her old friend Jimmy Hickey from the Dingle Glens with whom she used to flirt while travelling to work in the United States as a girl of eighteen. He still had a soft spot for her and on his return he had asked Pats Tom to keep an eye out for her so that they could meet again.

Méiní noticed that the people from the mainland used to make fun of the islanders as they walked in single file through the streets of Dingle or on the country roads. This habit was acquired because of the narrow pathways on the island and was strong enough to persist even when no longer necessary.

Another diversion within the island year were the special Masses held in the schoolhouse when a priest happened to be visiting. This was a frequent event in the summer as many of the younger priests were enthusiastic about the Irish language. The really big occasion was, however, the Station Mass. Tomás Ó Criomhthain describes the arrival of 'God's messengers'. An announcement would be a made by the priest at Sunday Mass in Dunquin that the islanders were to collect him on a certain day, and he would arrive on the island at about seven o'clock in the morning. The islanders were in their Sunday best, shaved and spruce as if they had never known a poor day. All the islanders had to do was to prepare the food which the priest brought with him. Méiní confessed that she had never noticed such a change among the Dunquin people as that among the islanders for the Station Mass. Young and old would gather on the cliffs, their hearts 'widening out' with welcome for the priest. 'On such an occasion,' she says, 'I had no regret that I slipped away from my own mother with a man from the island.'

Even when the weather was fine it was possible for only a small group of islanders to cross over regularly for Sunday Mass. While Mass was in progress in Dunquin, the older women would sit on a patch of green sward known as 'Máire Eoghain's bank'. It was called after the old woman, mother to 'Bell' Dunlevy, who was notable among those who used to gather there. From this vantage point they would look towards Dunquin while one of their number would lead them in saying the Rosary. In Méiní's day, the leaders in this group were Nelly Jerry, wife of Peats Tom Kearney, Máire Phats Mhicí, daughter of the King and wife to Mike Léan Guiheen and Kate Foley, from the mainland at Fahan, who was married to Séamus Stephen Dunlevy, the son of the Máire Eoghain who gave the bank its title.

Méiní and Seán Eoghain were not long married when another aspect of religion was dramatically demonstrated. They decided to start selling porter, and Willie Long of Ballyferriter, who was already selling flour and Indian meal to Méiní's mother, became their supplier – 'a pleasant straight man'. The police did not interfere with their trade, a fact which Méiní attributed to an understanding – bribery was the word she used – between Willie and the local police sergeant. The trade had continued for some time when the power of another law was made clear in the person of a visiting priest from England who was staying in the King's house. Unfortunately there was a nice sheltered little cubbyhole beside the King's house which was used by courting couples after dark on the summer evenings, and the priest's bedroom window overlooked this very spot. Méiní approved of the activity going on among those whose nature it was to be thus inclined: 'We were all like that,' she said, 'when our years of frolicsomeness and airiness of heart were on us, and it isn't right for priest or brother to be too hard on the natural inclinations of youth.' The priest took a markedly less liberal view, especially when those natural inclinations assumed an alcoholic hue. The young romantics, comfortably and regularly ensconced in their little den, did not realise that they were being watched. Méiní says that the priest never lit a light in his bedroom and was thus able to eavesdrop on the unfortunate young people without fear of detection, but one must say in his favour that she was not an unbiased informant.

The priest held his counsel until his holiday was over, and then wrote to the parish priest, Fr Griffin, appointed in 1906, detailing the undesirable behaviour of the young people of the island and emphasising how much of it was attribut-able to the effects of strong drink obtained at the shebeen. The very next Sunday, after Mass, Fr Griffin had himself rowed to the island. 'It doesn't matter what you see,' was Méiní's comment on what happened next, 'provided you don't see a priest angry with you!' No man or woman was left without a stern warning against drink and its evils; from that day onwards Méiní never sold another drop. Her comments in old age were restrained: 'We were not grateful to that priest, I can tell you!', but one would give much to have been a fly on the wall of the little house in the lower village when the parish priest had been safely rowed away and Seán Eoghain could express himself with all the vigour of his accustomed invective.

Méiní's neighbour, Paid Thomáis Kearney, son of 'Bald Tom', also ran a shebeen on the island at an earlier period.

We have met this eccentric and unpopular figure earlier in our story and it is hard to imagine him as a successful agent for a mainland supplier. His mother was Eileen Foley, the *cailleach bhéal dorais* (the old hag over the way) – of whom Ó Criomhthain wrote so scathingly. Tomás's description of her may just possibly have been a punning reference to the nickname of the Fahan Foleys, which was *coileach* (rooster) the two words resembling each other particularly with the Munster emphasis on the final syllable.

Though Méiní's shebeen had a short life, supplies of drink were not lacking while a sizable population remained on the island. A story has been recorded of some hardened topers from Dingle who decided to spend a weekend in the island where, they imagined, they would be free of temptation to indulge. Unfortunately, such were the island's resources, they returned home in far worse condition than on their arrival. But we must not lay the blame for that at Méiní's door.

11

MIDWIFE TO THE ISLAND

Although Méiní's vibrant personality and taste for fun ensured that, once her acquaintance was made, she was not easily forgotten, and although she was gifted as a storyteller, it was as midwife to the island community that she made her mark. Her contribution in this respect is mentioned in several places by writers about the Blaskets. An account of her work forms the initial section of Máire Guiheen's tale of *An tOileán a Bhí* (The Island That Was), and we shall learn that Máire herself was brought into the world with Méiní's help.

Several strands of experience served to direct Méiní towards her work as a midwife. Her grandmother Méireas was knowledgeable about herbal medicine and folk healing; we have already seen how Peig Sayers brought her young son to be cured of a fungal infection of the throat. She also had a cure for sprained ankle which consisted of binding the affected part with a cloth which had been boiled in a saucepan with the root and stem of wild comfrey. Although Méireas may never have cured anyone afflicted by 'overlooking' (the evil eye) she certainly passed on to her granddaughter an interest in such things, and showed her the herb called *luibh a' chiorraithe* which was used as a charm against and a cure for its baleful effects. Her mother Máire seems to have been less interested in such things than Méireas was but this was of little consequence to Méiní as, with the exception of her few years in America, she spent the years of her life up to her marriage in very close contact with her grandmother. This contact was maintained on her visits from the Blaskets for another twenty years until Méireas's death in 1917.

Within Dunquin itself there was a strong tradition of midwifery which may have stimulated Méiní's interest and was a direct source of her knowledge of the art. Ten minutes walk from her home, in the townland of Ballinaraha, lived Nell Pheig Fitzgerald who was for years the resident midwife to the Dunquin area. To the north of the parish in Ferriter's Quarter the family of Mitchell produced two midwives who lived and worked on the Blaskets, Cáit Shilbhí Mitchell, daughter of Silvester Mitchell and wife of Seán Mhichíl Kearney, and Nell Mhicil, daughter of Micil Mitchell, married to Maurice Paddy Keane. Also in Ferriter's Quarter lived Joanie Horgan, renowned for her skills in the parishes around. She was married to a tailor called Scanlon who spent regular spells on the island and their daughter Máire Scanlon helped Méiní in the middle years of her work.

During Méiní's early years on the island, when the doctor would arrive for difficult births or to carry out inoculation programmes, Cáit O'Brien, wife of Eoghan Bán O'Connor the weaver, would be called in to act as interpreter. Before her marriage she had worked with a doctor in Tralee and it is likely that English was her home language. At this stage Méiní would certainly have been able to speak English at least as well as Irish. Not only had she spent three years in America but prior to her marriage she was a frequent visitor to the O'Connor household in Ballinaraha who spoke English among themselves. On the island she frequently talked English to Máire Criomhthain, and was thus quite competent to take over the interpreting work at the request of the elderly Cáit. In this way she would have become known to the visiting dispensary doctors and to have been in a good position to pick up tips for her future profession.

Between the birth of Séamus in 1897 and that of Máire in 1903, Méiní lost several children in birth or early infancy and this stimulated her interest in the art of safe childbirth. Nell Mhicil Mitchell was the semi-official midwife on the island at the time of Méiní's arrival but she lived with her family in the Upper Village. Right next door to Méiní lived Seán Mhichíl Kearney and his wife Cáit Shilbhí. Possibly Cáit had worked as a midwife before marrying into the island, or gathered some knowledge of the art from helping Nell Mhicil who was a relative of hers. Méiní always claimed that it was her neighbour who stimulated her interest and taught her most of what she knew. Cáit's daughter had married on the island in 1899, and a son and another daughter in 1901, so her grandchildren were being born in Méiní's early years on the island. Cáit was in all likelihood present at many of these births, and may have brought Méiní as an interested neighbour to help on these occasions.

Méiní has given two separate accounts of how she first took responsibility for the management of an island birth. She gave one to Mike Pheig Sayers, but the following, largely in her own words, comes from a tape she made with me in 1962.

Nell Mhicil was getting old – she was the old nurse they had in the island at that time. I would be helping her when anyone would be sick until in the end I was taking most of the weight off the old woman. In the end, the old woman wasn't able to come for anyone. A woman came to her time and it wasn't possible to go out for the doctor because the weather was too bad to make the crossing. When he saw what the day was like Seán Eoghain said to me: 'Méiní, wouldn't you be able to give any help to Máire 'Lís?'

'Holy Mother!' I said, 'what would I do?'

''Tis all the same,' he said, 'perhaps Nell Mhicil will come with you.' Up I gets and off with me to Máire 'Lís and I didn't call at all on Nell Mhicil. 'Twasn't long before a young son was born to Máire – that's the man we call today Mike White. Michael O'Shea, her husband, was full of pride. And to think that his wife was well and flourishing.

The mother in that story was an O'Sullivan whose brother Seán was the father of Maurice O'Sullivan, author of *Twenty Years A-Growing*.

Though it was he who suggested that Méiní would go to help Máire, Seán Eoghain had no intention of allowing his young wife to neglect him by doing anything more in that line:

'Now I'm putting an end to all that,' said my own man to me. 'That'll be the end of your going out to any other woman. They can chose another old woman for themselves.'

'Indeed it won't be the end,' I answered him. 'I'd never do the like. Not from the moment when God gave me the knowledge to do it. I would give relief to any person that I was able to give it to.'

And that, for the moment, was that.

Infant mortality was high on the island at this period as it was often impossible for reason, amongst others, of bad weather, for the dispensary doctors to reach the island quickly enough in the case of difficult births. The island midwives knew enough to cope with ordinary cases, although the sanitary conditions were often dangerous and few attempts were made to give real professional training to an island nurse. On one occasion Dr Murphy came to the island to attend the confinement of Gobnait Kennedy. Since Gobnait was married in 1911 the visit in question must have been nearly twenty years after Méiní's arrival when she would have been in her late thirties. Dr Murphy had to stay overnight in the island and Méiní helped him with the birth. In the morning he said to Méiní that he would give her her paper and that she would get fifty pounds a year as a retainer.

'Oh I couldn't do that, doctor,' Méiní cried, 'I'd have to go to Dublin and I couldn't do that at all.'

'You won't have to do that,' said the doctor. 'I'll give a certificate at the courthouse that you are able to look after mothers better than any of the nurses that have learning. Don't I see you at your work? Get your paper tomorrow from Nack (Seán Dónal Kavanagh, father of Kruger, who lived in Ballinaraha and seems to have performed some of the functions of a peace commissioner) and bring it into the boardroom and I'll be there to meet you. Don't put in fifty pounds; if you put in forty-five you'll get forty but if you put in fifty you'll get forty-five.'

'Well, all that was fine and it certainly wasn't bad,' recalls Méiní, 'until I told my partner the story. I can tell you he was not one bit satisfied with me. He let a screech out of him: 'What would I be doing going out on the mainland with you?'

'Well, I'll go with the devil himself!' I said to him. 'I'll take my paper myself.'

'You will not take it and if you take it, it isn't here you'll be!' In the heel of the hunt I didn't return my paper to Nack or bring it to the boardroom to Dr Murphy. I never went back to Nack again. 'That was a good chance, 'tis a senseless woman you are!' said

Cáit Shilbhí to me. 'Méiní?' she said to me, 'wouldn't you take your chance?'

'I won't take it because it doesn't please my husband,' was all I could answer, and divil a word we ever spoke about the matter again.

Tomás Ó Criomhthain gives an account of the procedure at the birth of island children in *Allagar na hInise*. The midwife who delivered the child stayed with the mother until the morning and then took herself off to catch up on her own sleep. Tomás points out the extent to which a belief in the power of the fairies, or Good People, persisted in the island people of his day in spite of the abandonment of so many customs. For the first night after the birth of the child two old women had to be found to stay up for the whole night to make sure that the child was not stolen away. The fire blazed up through the night, food and drink were provided and lashings of tobacco to keep the old women's clay pipes burning until daylight. There was always an ample supply of whiskey on an occasion like this but it was never given to the old women lest they be fuddled with drink and the baby be stolen from under their noses in the dark. When the man of the house rose in the morning and the baby was seen to be still safe in the cot, the old women would be given a good big drop before setting off for their own homes. Needless to relate, the man of the house never forgot himself in the distribution.

Méiní told Mike Pheig Sayers that when she began to help old Nell Mhicil Mitchell with the island confinements their pay was half-a-crown (twelve and a half pence) and a good wedge of tobacco for their *dúidín*. She also told him how she first took responsibility for a birth and her story differs in every respect from that of her account of Mike White's birth.

She tells how her mother-in-law Máire Boland acted as

midwife in addition to Nell Mitchell, who had now given up through old age. One day when Máire Boland had gone to the mainland, Nell Kearney, who was the wife of Mike O'Sullivan, an uncle of Maurice, came into labour. None of the old women would come to the sick woman, but, Méiní says, she had the spirit to do it herself because her own mother had that trade. Since it does not appear that Máire Keating was at any time a midwife, Méiní is probably referring to her mother-in-law. She stayed with Nell Kearney until a young girl was born, and she was proud of this achievement because the birth was obviously a difficult one. Méiní had been with the mother for a while and told Nell's sister that she should send for the doctor. The sister went over to her own home where the baby's father was staying and he started to collect three or four men to man the *naomhóg* which would fetch help from the mainland. When the sister returned, Méiní told her to stop the crew leaving as there was nothing wrong with the baby. The girl who was born was 'Lís, named after her own, and Maurice O'Sullivan's, grandmother. In 1942 'Lís married into Kilmalkedar parish, a few miles from Dunquin.

One of Méiní's most amusing birth-stories concerns the birth of Máire Mhike Léan Guiheen, afterwards the wife of Labhrás Larry Ó Cíobháin, and author of two books about Blasket life. Méiní's own account is as follows:

There was a call to Dr Hudson to the island for Máire Guiheen who was ill in childbirth. Father Griffin, the parish priest, was in the island before him. The day was very bad and because of the tide that was running the priest had to be taken out of the boat at the 'Nune (the Blasket harbour) with the help of a rope. The doctor asked when the priest returned to the mainland if the harbour was suitable for going into the island. The priest said that it was and that he

94

knew the woman would not bring the child to birth without his help. He came to the island and he and the boat had to be pulled up on the slip at the harbour, the sea and the pull of it were so strong. He came up to the sick woman's house. The house was full of women and he himself was soaked from the sea. There was a nice sweet little woman there, Máire Mhuiris Keane, wife of Tom Kearney. 'My pity on you, doctor!' she said. 'You're all drowned wet.' The woman was rubbing the doctor dry and he shouted at her in English. 'May the divil take you! You wouldn't rub the best part of me!'

'Don't be in any hurry, doctor!' I said, because I had English and no one had English on the island at that time. We went to the room where the sick woman was lying and he went to work on her. I was with him to help. We weren't long there till he brought a young daughter into the world for Máire Guiheen. We settled her down, and he was exhausted, the poor man. He went to his big overcoat and there was a drop of brandy in the pocket. He told me to give him a wineglass. I asked the sister Cáit, she's the Princess now, if she had a small glass and of course she had. He filled the glass and he drank it down. He was putting the cork back in the head of the bottle to put it back in his pocket. 'God blast you!' said Méiní, 'Aren't you going to give me any drop?'

'I will,' he said, 'if you'll take it!' He jammed the bottle to my head and poured down my throat all that was in it until I put my tongue out against the drink. He put it back then into his pocket and sat down on a chair. He put tobacco in his pipe and smoked his fill. 'Yerra, doctor,' said the nurse (that was myself), 'Aren't you going to give me any smoke?'

'I will,' he said, 'if you'll take it.' He threw the

tobacco out of the pipe, and after he filled it again I smoked my fill of it. I did the same with the tobacco; I banged it out on my fist. 'May the divil carry you!' he said. 'What did you do with my tobaccy?'

'You saw what I did, doctor. You didn't give me your leavings and I didn't want to give you mine.'

'May the divil carry you! You're like the woman that Aristotle tells about because you have a woman's mind as quick as two men!'

We were very satisfied, and the sick woman was doing very well. There was a nice fire up in the kitchen, and I said to Máire Scanlon to come down to the room with me. The doctor wanted to warm himself at the fire. There were two beds in the room and the tick was rolled up on the other bed. Máire came down and stretched out on the bed nice and comfortable on her back. I went up to the kitchen. 'God bless you now, doctor!' I said. 'Come down to the room till you see Máire Scanlon.' He went down to the room and went up to the sick woman. 'How do you feel now?' he said. 'I'm good now, doctor,' was her answer. He turned around to come down again to the kitchen fire. He saw Máire and the cut of her on the bed. He stretched himself flat on Máire who let out terrible screeches, calling for help to take the doctor off her. He wouldn't let go the grip he had of her until Peggy Flint (Peig Sayers's sister-in-law) put the point of a big pin through one cheek of his backside – that was the time he let go his grip on Máire. He gave the brandy to the sick woman, and watched her as she was drinking it. He asked her how she felt. 'Very good, little doctor,' she said, stroking his face because of the relief he had given her. 'Look,' he said, 'all the women are fond of me but the men aren't!'

The birth recounted here took place in June 1909. During the years straddling the start of the century the Dingle dispensary doctors were John F. M. Miles, an Edinburgh graduate, and Robert Hudson, a licentiate in medicine of TCD. Hudson was a licentiate in midwifery, in contrast to Miles, so that to him fell most of the emergency trips to the Blaskets. His eye for the ladies, which may well have been exaggerated by his unsophisticated island friends, meant that there was usually a certain amount of fun while he was there, and he remained firmly in the memory and affection of the older islanders.

Some time after his arrival in 1906 the wife of the new teacher, Thomas Savage, was expecting a baby and Nell Mhicil Mitchell, assisted by Máire Scanlon, was acting as midwife. Mrs Savage did not have a word of Irish at that time and the midwife had next to no English. As Méiní recalled to Mike Pheig Sayers, 'When she would tell them to do this or that they used to do the wrong thing.' The upshot, again in Méiní's words, was that 'again I was sent for, and if I was, it wasn't I that would give the refusal. We did what was needed with the help of God. After that, when the doctor came, I used to be with him.'

From the early years of the century, therefore, until just after she left the island around 1933, Méiní was involved in one capacity or another at the birth of the island children. The families during this period tended to be large even when one counts only the children who survived birth and early infancy. Among the children at whose births she assisted were the families of 'Buffer' (Michael Keane, a brother of the King), and Mike Léan Guiheen; among the Kearneys were the numerous offspring of Pats Tom, Seán Tom, Filí, Séasaí and the *Poncán*. In her later years on the island, when Nell Mhicil and Cáit Shilbhí were no more, Méiní was assisted not only by Máire Scanlon, but also by Gobnait Kennedy and these two women may have acted independently on occasion. Máire, as we have seen, was the daughter of the Dunquin midwife Joanie Horgan and had her house at the very top of the village near the well called after her husband.

The well was a natural place for the women to gather around as they waited for their buckets to fill, but Máire was in the centre of the island life for the further reason that her house was so often the scene of discussions and informal debates. From this fact the lady of the house was referred to as 'Máire of the *Dáil*' or 'Máire of the Tailor' after her father's profession. Hers was also a favourite house for the young folk of the island to gather in during the evenings for dancing and music. Máire's own family, all of whom left eventually for America, tended to attract the other young people. One of Máire's sons, Thomas, was born in the year that Méiní married.

Gobnait Kennedy was a much younger woman and a close friend and neighbour of Méiní. She was married to Pats Shéamuis Guiheen, son of the Pat Shéamuis who figures so largely in *An tOileánach* because he was married to the author's sister. She was better known as a storyteller than as a midwife. Examples of her style may be found in Robin Flower's *The Western Island* in which a translation of her version of the tale of Purty Deas Squarey is given, one among many which he recorded. (We reproduce a fine photograph showing Méiní and Gobnait together. Méiní can be seen with her two hands locked together over her stomach, a pose which she liked to adopt when being photographed, right into her last years.)

The last Blasket birth at which Méiní is known to have assisted occurred around the year 1933, in the first months of her widowhood when she had left the island. Máiréad Kavanagh from Ventry was married to Seán Keane, son of the king of the island who had died about four years earlier. 'Mag an Rí' as she was called, came into labour and her husband, who had succeeded his father as island postman, made the double crossing with Paddy Shéasaí Kearney and Seán Mhike Léan Guiheen to bring back Méiní. They used the mainland cove at Fáill Chliadh which was the original Dunquin harbour and nearer to Méiní's house. All went well and Mag was delivered of a girl. Unfortunately, the father Seán had only a year to live as he died in 1934 of blood poisoning.

Settled back in Dunquin, Méiní continued her work for a year or two. Mícheál Mistéal of Ballinahow, then a child of about seven, clearly remembers her coming for the birth of his sister Kathleen.

12

SORROW ON THE SEA

Because of her experience in the life-and-death situations associated with many of the births on the isolated island, Méiní was called on to cope with the tragedies which inevitably arise among communities which earn their living from the sea. In the years when she lived there, the island community never numbered more than about one hundred and sixty people and, given the fact that six or seven families had seven or eight children, the actual number of family units was small and intermarriage between the families was considerable. For that reason, any tragedy would involve personal or family grief for an appreciable proportion of the islanders and in varying degrees for the whole village: 'When one of our people would be drowned or would fall suddenly over a cliff, that's what would be a terrible disturbance and misfortune to us all.'

The first such incident of which Méiní has left a record concerns the double drowning on 13 August 1909 of Eveleen Nicolls from Dublin, and Dónal Ó Criomhthain, son of Tomás, off the White Strand. The story has been told many times and is the subject of an extensive study by Mícheál Ó Dubhshláine. Eveleen Nicolls was a graduate of University College Dublin in Celtic Languages and came from a well-to-do Dublin family. Her interest in the Irish language had brought her into contact with Patrick Pearse and it has been said that there was an 'understanding' between them.

The precise details of the drownings are confused and the different accounts are difficult to reconcile. Nevertheless, the main outlines are clear. Eveleen had gone for a swim at the White Strand at high water around two in the afternoon accompanied by the Princess, that is Kate Keane, daughter of the king of the island, at whose house she had been staying for five weeks. On the way to the beach they called for Kate Criomhthain, Tomás's daughter, to whom Eveleen had been giving swimming lessons and were joined there by Máire Keane. The Princess had a cold and did not go swimming with the other three. For some reason Kate Criomhthain got into difficulties and Eveleen swam to her assistance but she herself became exhausted and sank. Kate Keane was watching and seeing that something was wrong shouted for help. She heard Eveleen shouting her name and bravely entered the water fully clothed. Dónal Ó Criomhthain heard the Princess's shouts for help, rushed to the beach, dragged the Princess herself from the sea and swam out in his clothes and boots to rescue Eveleen. In the meantime, Máire Keane had got ashore and was helping to raise the alarm. Pats Tom Kearney entered the water as soon as he arrived at the strand and was able to keep Kate Criomhthain afloat and finally to bring her ashore. Most of the men were at the fishing grounds and there was considerable delay in getting a *naomhóg* manned and over to the White Strand.

Dónal Ó Criomhthain may or may not have reached Eveleen in his rescue attempt but by the time their bodies were recovered, life was extinct. One report says that the first boat on the scene was able to help Pats Tom Kearney in rescuing Kate Criomhthain but one would imagine that it was unlikely to have arrived on time. The second boat to arrive located the body of Dónal Ó Criomhthain and brought it ashore. The third boat on the scene had on board Fr Jones from Glenbeigh who had come on a day trip, and the crew, which included Méiní's step-son Eoghan, set about finding Eveleen's body. There was considerable delay in finding this as the ebb tide had moved it farther along the shoreline. In the meantime, Pats Tom Kearney had joined the third boat and lifted Eveleen's body from the water. This basic account was given by James Cousins of Dublin, poet, dramatist, Irish enthusiast and spiritualist, and published in the *Cork Constitution* a few days later. He had come across to visit Eveleen and was accompanied by Fionán Mac Coluim, chief Munster organiser of the Gaelic League. They reached the slip at the island harbour as the boat was bringing in the body of his friend amid the shouts and the excitement.

Méiní was called on to prepare the bodies of Eveleen and Dónal for coffining and she reminisced about the drowning on many occasions. My own record of what she said dates from 1957 and differs in some respects from that given to Mike Pheig Sayers about the same time. She first noticed that something was amiss when, standing at her door, she saw Dónal Ó Criomhthain, who had earlier been taking produce to the pier, running past through a field of potatoes. According to her, the men in the boat took two hours to find Eveleen's body which they finally retrieved with a hook on the end of an oar. At the pier, when the body was brought ashore, Fr Jones asked Méiní for hot water. She got this from a neighbour who was preparing dinner and Eveleen's body was rubbed with it in an attempt to revive her. Dónal's body must have been lying nearby. Méiní maintained that Peig Sayers tried to have more attention paid to the island boy and that Máire Mhuiris, wife of Tom Kearney, said angrily: 'Why shouldn't we save the poor man's son?' At this point, according to the story, Fr Jones took umbrage, and, turning around asked, 'Who said that?' On receiving no answer he turned around again and said, 'Who said that?' And again a third time he asked: 'Who said that?' When as yet he received no answer he gave up his attempts to revive Eveleen.

Here we can see clear signs that Méiní's memory was getting confused and her natural gift for storytelling was taking over and moulding events into a traditional narrative form. Plainly Fr Jones gave up his attempts when they were obviously futile such a long time after the drowning, but in the intervening half-century a slightly sinister element had insinuated itself into the account. This element is lacking in the story which Méiní gave to Mike Pheig Sayers, or perhaps his natural piety may have led him to omit it if she mentioned it to him. She said that after the drowning she never liked to be alone on the White Strand; she often thought that the waves there were lamenting Eveleen and the young man who gave his life on her behalf.

Dónal's body was brought to his own home for the wake and Eveleen's body was brought to the King's house where she had been lodging. Kruger Kavanagh has told how his brother 'Seán a' Chóta' had arrived on the island with Fr Jones as he was also a friend of Eveleen who had stayed at his home in Ballinaraha. To Kruger himself fell the task of running in his bare feet to Ventry to send to Eveleen's parents on Rathgar Road the telegram which Fr Jones had dictated. 'Seán a' Chóta' supervised the funeral which was the biggest ever seen in Dunquin up to that time, and was attended, according to local tradition, by Patrick Pearse himself.

Méiní's nephew, Martin Keane, remembered clearly the two coffins arriving at Dunquin pier, a very dramatic event for a young boy. He also remembered hearing that Tomás Ó Criomhthain received about one pound a week from the Nicolls family from that time onward in recognition of his son's bravery in going to Eveleen's rescue. Tomás acknowledges their kindness to him in a moving way: 'The lady's family were very kind to me for years afterwards. They both came, the father and the mother, to see me in Dunquin and had me pointed out to them. I hope they did not think I was angry with them because my son had died for their daughter.'

The tradition that Pearse came to Dunquin for Eveleen's funeral must be treated with some caution, as it would have been more natural for him to have attended the burial in Dublin. Séamus 'Twoee' Kavanagh has said that he saw Patrick Pearse at a féis organised by Tomás Ághas and others on the cliff in Dunquin in 1912. Séamus's memory was demonstrably strong on dates and Pearse's visit to Dunquin might easily have become attached in local memory to the funeral three years earlier.

Some twenty years before Dónal was drowned, Tomás's eldest son had been killed on the cliffs when birds-nesting. Eleven years after the drowning he was getting mussels to manure his field for an early potato crop when another son ran up to tell him that Peig Sayers's son Tomás had fallen down a cliff. When pulling a tuft of gorse for the fire he had toppled backwards and had plunged to the rocks below. Peig was shattered by this death, especially so since her husband's health was failing fast. In her later years she often spoke about this time to her grandniece Máire, now Bean Uí Lúing, who has a clear recollection of these conversations.

A sense of awe hit the people of the island at this tragic death, so much so that many were afraid to stay in the house with the unfortunate woman, even her own children being reluctant to come in. 'When they came in,' Máire reports, 'they wouldn't stay inside but off with them immediately except for one woman only and that was Méiní.' She used to say to Peig, 'Keep up your courage, girl, and God will help you. You will have help from the Virgin Mary to go through all this.'

'But Méiní,' said the distracted mother, 'it is very hard on me and I don't think I'll ever be able to get through it, especially as the poor boy's father is a terrible care for me as I don't know the minute he will leave me.'

Méiní went up to the schoolhouse where Mass was celebrated and brought down to Peig's house the statue of the Virgin which stood there. This gave her heart to go through those times. The body of the unfortunate boy had been laid on the floor of Peig's house. As a result of the fall from the cliff he had received appalling head injuries. Méiní and the distracted mother bound up his shattered skull as best they could with makeshift bandages. His back was broken and – a strange detail that his mother recalled – his hand was in his pocket.

Because of the heavy seas and storms there was delay in bringing the body to the quay at Dunquin, and the father, Patsy Flint, was so weak that he was barely able to walk the short distance from his bed to pay his respects to his son's body. Peig feared that it might be two bodies that would cross the Blasket Sound. She prayed to the statue of the Virgin to grant a change in the weather, and the funeral procession of *naomhóga*, some of them from Dunquin, was eventually able to set off on the journey to the family burial place at Ventry from which the Sayers family had come in Peig's father's time.

Peig herself did not attend the burial of her son; she felt that her first duty was to remain to look after her dying husband. It was a fortnight before her two daughters Cáit and Nell could summon up the courage to come home to her, such a shock had they received on seeing the body of their brother. During all this time, Méiní ministered to the broken woman. The manner in which she enabled her to preserve her sanity and fortify her religious faith in those dark times was never forgotten by Peig until her dying day.

13

Stories and Storytelling

This is not the place and I do not have the necessary expertise to attempt a full-scale study of Méiní as a storyteller. Nonetheless not to deal with this aspect of Méiní's life is unthinkable. I am however confining my account and the examples I give to those stories I myself recorded from her at her home in Ballykeen, Dunquin, during the years 1956 to 1963 when she was over eighty years of age. In a few cases I know of other versions of the same stories recorded from Méiní herself, and the comparison between the versions would provide material for scholarly treatment. In such cases I have confined myself to my own version.

In Méiní's lifetime, although her stories were enjoyed by many people who visited her, she had none of the acclaim as a *seanchaí* which was earned by Peig Sayers, and to some extent by Gobnait Kennedy. We have already noted that in *The Western Island* Flower tells of a visit made to the house of Seán Eoghain and Méiní, and of how they were joined by Gobnait, who on this occasion was definitely the star. Méiní's sole function, apart from an occasional interjection, was to wet the tea and to light the candle. It is generally accepted that, at least on the Blaskets, Peig Sayers was in a class of her own, but the amount of surviving material from

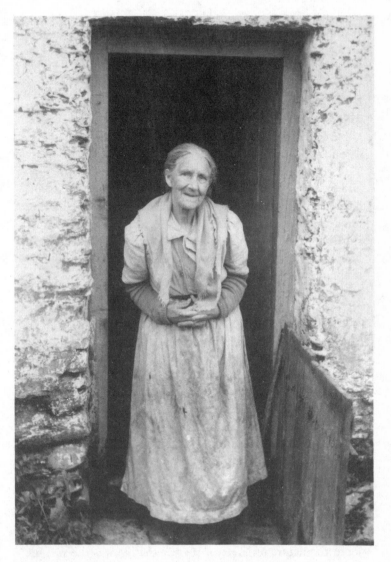

Méiní, aged 82. The dog has his own half-door.

Méiní, when adequately studied, may well increase her posthumous status.

Some of Méiní's stories have been taken down by amateur enthusiasts, but the bulk of those which survive are in the archives of the Irish Folklore Commission. Many of these were obtained by trained collectors such as Dr Joe Daly, who was brought up a few fields away from Méiní's Dunquin home. Appended to the account of her life which Méiní gave to Mícheál Pheig Sayers is a collection of some one hundred and thirty stories of varying lengths which he took down from her.

Two particular problems arise in connection with this latter group of stories. Many of them are accounts of happenings involving persons of earlier generations right up to Méiní's own time. Some purists feel that to dignify such stories with the title of folklore is to confer on them too honourable a status. I am not qualified to comment on this judgement except to say that in recent years a more comprehensive meaning seems to be applied to the term. Greater importance is now being attached to the recording of contemporary and near-contemporary happenings, beliefs and life-patterns.

Another caveat should be entered in relation to the stories recorded by Mícheál. He says that he took down the stories in an old account book and complains of the labour involved in transcribing them into the fair copies which were then dispatched to Dublin. It is therefore not possible, in the absence of the original notes, to judge to what extent he added his own adjustments and glosses to what he took down from Méiní's lips. He was a considerable storyteller in his own right, with a strong sense of the importance of accuracy and the maintenance of a literary flavour. Having heard him argue somewhat abrasively with Méiní's nephew Martin about the nature of poetry, I suspect that he was the sort of man who may have been tempted to improve on the versions given him. We may never know for certain.

Though Mícheál was not a purist in the sense that we can be confident that he preserved all the narrative and grammatical features of the stories he recorded, there is ample evidence that he was puritan by nature. I do not think that Méiní yielded anything to the *File* in the sincerity of her religious faith, which in both was patent, but I believe she had a taste for the risqué story which he may well have enjoyed but would have hesitated to commit to writing. Indeed, her own daughter, Máire Kilcoyne, in a recording made in 1962, chides Méiní for introducing a suspect element into a story, a charge which she rebuffs.

The years during which Mícheál was writing down Méiní's stories coincided with the years when I had closest contact with her. It was obvious to me that Méiní regarded him with a certain mild antagonism, and on one or two occasions she said to me, 'I didn't give this story to the *File* as I was keeping it for you.' The source of her suspicion was in no way related to any feeling that he was doctoring what she was telling; such a mode of thinking would have been quite foreign to her experience. Mícheál had a reputation for generosity in many small ways, particularly to children, but, having a somewhat touchy manner, he was not generally popular in Dunquin. His high estimate of the value of the poet's calling led him to refuse social welfare assistance, at least for some time. This may have created the impression of a certain intellectual snobbery, but in Méiní's case, she felt that he was making a good thing out of her stories because it was known that he was being paid for those he transmitted to Dublin.

The point has been made that the best storytellers on the Blaskets were in fact blow-ins of mainland origin. Tomás Ó Criomhthain's father had come as a young man from Ballykeen in Dunquin, Peig was from Baile Bhiocáire, Gobnait Kennedy hailed from the Gortha Dubha and Méiní belonged to a Dunquin family with Iveragh connections.

Too much can be made of these facts. In the first place many of those who were third and fourth generation islanders did not have their stories recorded, to some extent because they were less at ease with strangers than those accustomed to mainland life. The crucial point is that all the Blasket islanders were of relatively recent mainland origin, as witness the number of families who returned to Ventry cemetery to bury their dead. I think that a better argument can fairly be made that the Blasket people deserve credit for providing the social structure and climate of appreciation which enabled storytelling talents to develop and flourish. In this connection, it may be noted that the hero-tales such as those of the Fenian warriors and of the Red Branch Knights were generally considered better adapted for telling by male storytellers, as were the fairy-tales for females, but this is a distinction which should not be pushed too far.

The short selection of stories is taken from the few I had the opportunity to record in writing and on tape, and chosen to give a varied selection illustrative of Méiní's concerns and interests. Although many of the details of her life were given to me in a mixture of Irish and English, her stories were entirely in Irish and translated by me direct from the notebooks in which I took them down over thirty years ago. At some points, local idiosyncrasies of pronunciation and vocabulary caused me difficulty, armed as I was with little more Irish than I had learned at school. I do not pretend to have ironed out all the problems, and I give preference to stories in which these occur least. I have related them as far as possible to the unfolding story of Méiní's life.

In the early chapters, I have told how Bridget Keating brought her son Seán from the Iveragh peninsula at Ballinskelligs towards the middle of the nineteenth century. This first story may well relate to the family of Bridget's husband, Méiní's great-grandfather. It has elements which interested Méiní as a midwife, and also reflects the great hospitality which was given to beggars in Dunquin, none more so than by her grandmother Méireas Emperor. It is a simple story, illustrative of the heartlessness and kindliness which mingles uneasily in the experience of the dependent poor.

There was a couple in Iveragh, Nell Keating was the girl's name and Séamus Hassett was the boy's. The girl's family did not want her to marry Séamus but her love was so strong that she wouldn't marry any man except him. She and Séamus married in spite of her people. She was married a year when Séamus her husband died. His people fought with her and they put her out of the house. When she came home to her own people's house, her father and mother put her out also. She went to the house of an aunt of Séamus who left her stay until morning. She went away the next day, the poor girl, begging for a living. She was married well over the nine months at the time.

She went into Ned Power's house in Listowel; it was Christmas Eve night. She asked to be let in until the day. They refused her – they had eaten the supper and the candle was lit when she had to go away. There was a poor house on the corner before her, Tim Leahy's house. The supper was ready just at the moment when she asked them would she be let into the house until the morning.

'That will be allowed,' said the woman of the house, 'and a thousand welcomes. Tonight is Christmas Eve, the night on which the Son of God was given to us.'

They let her in and she got the big supper they

had themselves. It wasn't long after Nell had finished the supper that she started to suffer pain and sickness.

'Oh Holy Mother!' said Siobhán, the woman of the house, to Tim. 'Would you go out to Neligan's house to tell Bridie to come?'

Bridie came in and spoke to the sick girl. 'What's wrong, girl?' she asked. 'I think it's going into labour I am.'

Bridie went home and told the news to Denis her husband.

'What job did Siobhán have for you?' he enquired.

'It was the poor girl that's inside with her,' she replied. 'She's going to have a baby, Denis,' she said. 'I'm going to bring her in here, if you agree with me.'

'I'd do the same myself,' he said, 'if only I'd know who'd be in need of being left in.'

They took her in to their own home and the man of the house went out to get the doctor for her. They treated her in a very friendly way, and when the doctor came he said to her:

'Good girl,' he said, 'where did you get that baby?'

'Oh, doctor,' she said, 'it wasn't behind the ditch that I got it but I was married. I was married half a year when my partner died. I was carrying the baby then and my husband's people threw me out. My own people put me out also and I had to take to the road. That big house down there,' she said. 'I asked them to leave me in until dawn. It was Christmas Eve but I had to turn into a poor couple's house. There was no lack of welcome for me no more than from the couple I'm with now. May God grant them prosperity!'

A young son was born to her, and she called him Séamus after his father. The man of the house kept her as a servant girl and they took her child and gave him schooling until he was sixteen years of age. His mother and himself were working until they came back to Iveragh, where they lived happily ever after.

Growing up in Dunquin, Méiní would have seen the little boys of her own age wearing girls' dresses, and would have known that this was to deceive the 'little people' – the fairies – into thinking that they were girls, whom fairies were not disposed to steal. For the same reason, boys were very often called by nicknames to conceal their identity from them. As Seán Ó Súilleabháin has written (*A Handbook of Irish Folklore*, 1942), 'It is very difficult to draw a clear line of demarcation between the kingdom of the dead and the fairy world.' The story which follows, about a mainland girl, exemplifies this to some extent, and is attractive in its simple blending of contemporary life and activity with the supernatural world.

There was a little girl in Ballymore – a schoolgirl she was. When she came home from school one day, her mother asked her would she be agreeable to go to the post office to post a letter to her aunt who was in America. Bridie set off at half-past four for the post office – 'twas in Annascaul that the post was in those days. Bridie had twelve miles to go. The night had already fallen on her when she met a woman who was doing her washing in a river.

'Where are you going?' said the woman to Bridie.

'I'm going to the post office,' answered Bridie.

''Tis too late for you now,' said the woman. 'The first house you meet go inside and stay till morning.'

Bridie set off again and she met the house by the roadside. She went in and there was an old person inside putting a fine pot of potatoes on the fire.

'God bless you, Bridie Kennedy!' said the old man. 'Have you any news to tell me?'

'No, I haven't,' said Bridie.

She wasn't in the house long when a sheep came up from the back room. The sheep was wearing a white apron. Bridie's eyes were popping out of her head when she saw the sheep with the apron on her. The sheep took down the pot, drained the potatoes and threw them out on a bit of cloth on the table. Bridie was watching the sheep when all this was going on. The sheep gave her butter and milk along with the potatoes. She ate the potatoes herself along with the old man. Then the sheep took the utensils off the table and when that was done she made Bridie a cup of tea before she went to bed. When she had made the tea, the sheep went back to the lower room. She came back down the floor as a beautiful woman; she was no longer a sheep.

'There now, Bridie Kennedy,' said the old man, 'if you didn't have a new story coming, you'll have a new one going away!'

The two eyes were dazzled out of Bridie.

'Now,' said the woman that was a sheep, 'as long as you live again, let your mother not give you any job during the night. I'm your godmother, and I knew you'd be dead in the morning by the fairies!'

She arranged a bed in the corner for Bridie.

'Sleep your fill now,' she said.

When she woke in the morning, the sun was shining on Bridie. There was no house around her but herself sleeping on the rushes.

Bridie went to the post office and came back home again.

'What kept you out last night?' said her mother.

'Oh, what happened was that I met my godmother in the river and she kept me until morning, so now I have a new story to tell. It was a sheep that was boiling the food for us. In my opinion, that's the way it was.

There's a new story for you!'

From that day onwards after the day that she came home, she didn't delay on the road to Annascaul, but lived happily ever after.

This story illustrates a common theme of the adoption of human characteristics by animals. Living in a society that was so close to animals and so directly dependent on them, it was natural that Méiní should accept the supernatural role attributed to them in the fireside stories she heard. In many of the religious stories to be found throughout the country, the cock plays an important part, reflecting its Gospel role in the poignant story of the betrayal of Jesus by Peter. In one very jumbled story of Méiní's, the cock appears at one point with a different function:

Tim Crihin was living in Gortachlochair. He and his wife Kate lived alone. 'Tis how they used to say a prayer every Sunday; when Mass was on they used to say the Rosary at the same time.

One Sunday when he was indoors – Kate had gone to Mass – Tim started to say the Rosary. He was halfway through it when the cock came on to the frame of the door. He started crowing while Tim was praying.

'May God silence you!' he said to the cock who was crowing.

As soon as he said that to the cock, its soul fell out of it. When Tim rose from his prayers, he went out and looked up into the sky. There was a black cloud and Tim was filled with fear and terror. He said to himself that the cloud was coming to take the blessed cock away.

Well, Kate came home from Mass; Tim hadn't boiled either potatoes or fish.

'For God's sake!' said Kate. 'Didn't you put the potatoes boiling?'

'I didn't, Kate,' he said. 'I was saying my prayers and the cock came to the frame of the door and was crowing loudly. "May God silence you," I said to the cock. When I said that the soul fell from the cock. Look at the black cloud that's up above. I think it's watching me because of the shout I gave at the blessed cock.'

'I'd say that you're right,' said Kate, 'because the lights of Heaven have gone out ever since. They have power over good and evil.'

When Kate boiled the potatoes and they were after eating their dinner, she said: 'Put your two hands now before the priest. Tell him your story.'

Tim did this through and through, telling the priest that he had been saying the Rosary: 'When the cock came crowing on the doorframe he was interrupting my prayers and I said, "May God silence you!" to it. His soul fell out of him. When I rose up, 'tis how there was a black cloud in the sky, and it scared me.'

'Oh that's what it was, Tim! It's a good thing you came. You'll have to go nine Fridays to the chapel and say a good amount of prayers every Friday, until you have the nine Fridays finished.'

He did the nine Fridays, and he called to the priest on the last one.

'Woe to you,' said the priest, 'that you didn't leave the cock alone, because that cock was keeping harm from you. There's no danger for you from now on; it doesn't matter what you say or what you write and you'll be able to say your prayers. Don't speak out loudly, because it's to God Himself that you are talking at that time. It doesn't matter what will break in on you or what will call.'

So when Tim was saying his prayers, he wouldn't ever speak. The priest said that the time of Mass was a solemn time and the parish cock would be crowing during that time.

Well, Kate got a cock and the cock didn't crow. She got another cock, so she had two cocks, but neither of the two cocks crowed.

A cock never crowed on that gate ever afterwards.

In what appears to be part of a different story altogether, Méiní appends the story of two brothers who were turned into seals and only released by human intervention – a story of which many related versions are known.

Another story in which a cock appears was related by Méiní concerning John Garvey of the Old Hill. As there have been Garveys in Carhoo for many generations, it may concern this family. It is the only story I have taken down from Méiní for which she gives the source. She said she heard it from Tom Long at Baile Bhiocáire about fifty years ago, that is, about the year 1906. Méiní was a pipe smoker up to the end of her life, and no doubt at times could not afford a supply of tobacco for her *dúidín*. For this reason, she may have felt particular sympathy for the hero of the story. The lesson given by the cock is hardly calculated to meet with feminist approval. *Autres temps, autres moeurs.*

There was a couple on the Old Hill, John Garvey and Mary Kennedy their names. He was a farmer and a great man for smoking tobacco. One day he came in from the field and he told his wife to go to the shop to get him a plug of tobacco. He went out again to the field. The wife went to the shop but she didn't get the tobacco. When he came in from the field in the evening he told his wife to give him his tobacco.

'I won't give it to you because I did not get it,' she

117

replied.

'Give me the price of it then so that I can go to Ventry to get it.'

'Will you have your supper?' asked his wife.

'I won't have it until I come home.'

He set off on the road, and he didn't stop until he reached Ventry. He went into the shop and there was no tobacco to be had. He set off home and he met an old man on the road. The old man stretched out his pipe to him and he had his fill of pulls at it. He handed back the pipe to the old man, who said: 'Buy it from me now with your pay.' John put his hand in his pocket.

'Oh, the pay that I'm looking for,' said the old man, 'is prayers for the dead.'

'May God's blessing be on your soul,' said John, 'and on all your dead.'

The old man reddened the pipe again and handed it to him. He smoked his fill and handed it back to the old man: 'May God's blessing be on your soul and on all your dead.'

'Now,' said the old man, 'this is your pipe and it will never be empty. But don't tell anyone who gave it to you. My sins are now completely forgiven. Go home now and I'm going high up to Heaven.'

When John came home, he ate his supper and he was fully satisfied going to bed. He was home for a week when his wife asked him where he got the pipe. He didn't give her any account at all.

His wife went upstairs to bed and wouldn't get up to do the housework or anything else. He went out to the field in the morning. No dinner was prepared for him. He prepared dinner himself and when he had eaten it up, it started to rain. He threw food for the hens on the floor of the house. He had six hens and a cock. Two hens were fighting and the cock went in and separated them. Two other hens started fighting, and again the cock went in and separated them.

'I have six women on my hands,' said the cock, 'and I am keeping control of them, and you can't keep control of one single woman.'

'That's true,' said the husband.

He got hold of the stick and went up to the room. He turned down the bedclothes off his wife and beat her heavily with the stick. She screeched out to let her go and not to be killing her entirely. 'I'll be your servant,' she said, 'as good as I ever was!'

She got up, and I can vouch for it that she was as good a servant as ever she was. Her husband and herself lived very happily until the day when death divided them.

Not all smokers were granted such a happy ending, and Méiní vouched for the truth of one such:

There was a man living in Caheratrant named Dónal Walsh. He was short of tobacco and was cross with his cat and his dog, cranky because he had nothing to smoke. The messenger was not coming with the tobacco.

'Take it easy!' said his wife. 'The help of God is nearer than the door.'

'That's the door!' he said, going towards it. 'We're short of the help of God!'

He stood at the door and he fell down where he stood and died. There's no lie in that. I remember his people myself.

When Méiní went to live in the Blaskets in 1896, one of her earliest friends was Máire Criomhthain, the sister of

Tomás. To her Méiní always gave credit for having told her many of the stories she herself was to pass on. Although Máire was thirty-five years older than Méiní, two factors in particular caused them to appreciate each other's company. In the first place, they both spoke English fluently and were anxious to keep up their ability to do this by speaking it together. Secondly, they had both spent time in the United States. Born in 1841 Máire Dhónail married Mártan Keane, her second cousin, in 1862. Mártan, the third son of Paddy Mhártan, lived only a year after the marriage. According to her brother Tomás, Máire left a son with her own family and went off to America. She accumulated enough money to take legal action on her return to recover Mártan's share of the Keane property for her young son, around about the year 1866. In 1872 she married Mikil, son of the poet Michael O'Sullivan, (the first O'Sullivan to come to the island). This is the reason why Méiní sometimes refers to her as Máire Sullivan. Méiní did not make a practice of giving the source of her stories – with the exception of the story of John Garvey above – but it is likely that at least some of them were Máire's.

For one story which she enjoyed telling – and the two versions I know of differ in some respects – we can find the source in Méiní's own experience. Although she said in 1962 that it happened forty years before, my own preference is for an earlier date, when her stepsons were young boys and Séamus was as yet her only child, in other words during the early years of her marriage.

My partner was out one night and Maurice, Eoghan and Séamus were in the cottage. When Seán Eoghain came to bed he didn't shut the door of the room. At any rate we weren't asleep long in the night when something came under the bottom of the bed, letting every screech out of it. Seán Eoghain gave me a poke to get up.

'What's that?' I said.

The thing was going backwards and forwards from the bed to the other side, knocking loudly.

'Oh yes!' said Seán Eoghain, 'it's the devil himself! May God protect me!'

He didn't say: 'May God protect Méiní!' but he was only pleading for himself. I sat up and the knocking was still going on in the room.

'Would you get up!' he said.

'Wouldn't you get up yourself?' I answered him. 'You're on the outside!'

'Oh, I couldn't do that!' he said.

I lit the candle at the foot of the bed, and he was trembling all over at the ghost that was under the bed. In the end I got up and I looked in under the bed, and 'tis how the kitten was there with the jug stuck on its head and I suppose a drop of milk in it. It was going up and down the room, calling out because the jug was caught on its head. I got hold of the cat's tail.

'Get hold of the cat's backside,' I said to Seán Eoghain, 'so that we can see if we can get its head out of the jug.'

'I won't do it, because it's the divil himself!' he said.

He wouldn't catch the cat, he was so frightened that it was the Old Boy himself that was there, and that he'd be eaten by him. I got hold of the cat and I put its backside between my legs, and I gripped the jug and tried to pull its head free. No sooner did I pull the jug off its head than I let him loose on the floor and 'twas how the poor cat was delighted to get its head back safe and sound.

'Where is he now?' said Seán Eoghain. 'By my

soul, will you put him out the door!'

'On my soul, I won't put it out!' I answered. 'I'm going to sleep now and the divil take you! You wouldn't even ask God's blessing on Méiní but were only thinking of protecting yourself from the Old Boy!'

The next morning when Tomás Ó Criomhthain came over, he said: 'That was a heroic deed Seán Eoghain did last night!'

'May God's curse be on him!' I said. 'You, Seán Eoghain,' I said, turning to him, "tisn't even one glance itself that you gave at that cat!'

Another version of this story was given five years previously by Méiní, and taken down when I was present. It differs from the above in that it concerns Seán and Mary, and it is only at the end that it is revealed that it is a story from her own married life. Seán gives as his reason for not getting out of bed that he had no shift on him.

Méiní loved to tell stories of Blasket islanders of olden days, and she was particularly attracted to stories about those who had adventures with animals or natural forces. Mollín or Moll is the subject of what follows. She was the daughter of Seán Guiheen (Senior) from Inishvickillane and his wife Máire de Mórdha.

There was a woman on the island long ago whose name was Molly, and one fine evening she went to the hill to get a load of turf from Bun an Dúna. She was filling the turf on to the donkey and when she raised her head she saw a big black thing coming from the north-east. She was frightened because she never before saw such a thing as came over her head. She lowered her back and at that moment what fell on her but a big yellow hen that had been taken by the eagle. The eagle was abandoning the hen because it got a pain in its paw and so the hen fell away from him.

The eagle got vexed and went for Molly instead of the hen. In she went under the donkey's belly until the eagle went away from her towards the cliff. She filled the load on the donkey and she brought home the hen, who was not harmed except for the mark of the claws scratched along her back.

'By Christ, Moll,' said Diarmuid her husband when he came home, 'we'll have fine yellow chickens from that hen!'

The yellow hen was laying and hatching and she gave twelve yellow chickens. The women of the village were coming buying the yellow hens. Everyone on the island had yellow hens from Molly's hen.

The doctor had come to Máire Guiheen and he went up past Molly's door going to Mrs Guiheen's. At that very moment, Molly was giving food to the hens just as the doctor was going past. She drove them away. When he was finished with the sick woman he came to Molly's house and Diarmuid and she were there before him. He said to Molly, 'Where did you get that breed of hen?'

'Over on the hill we got it!' said Diarmuid. 'That hen fell from an eagle.'

The doctor bought a half-dozen of the chickens from Molly. He put all about the hen in the paper and found out from whom the eagle took the hen. It was from Liam Brennan of Ballyheigue that the hen was stolen by the eagle. Dr Crump remembered that breed of chicken. Nothing on the hill ever met Molly to give her a fright from that day on. She and her husband lived very happily ever afterwards.

The next story, about Tomás Aindrias, was written down in

Irish at Méiní's dictation in September 1960. It differs in many details from a similar story about Tomás Aindrias given to Mícheál Ó Gaoithin at the same period. The two versions deserve comparative study to establish which details are accurate and which have been modified through forgetfulness or design. The *File* may well have heard the story from his mother or others, and some of the emendations may have been an attempt to reconcile what Méiní told him with other versions.

I have not been able to establish the identity of Tomás and Nora but he may have been the brother of the Patrick Guiheen, son of Andrew Geehan and his wife Mary Connell, of the Blaskets, who was baptised at Christmas 1836. The story is a sympathetic account of the plight of some of the poorest people on the island around the time of the Famine and the generosity shown to their neighbours by at least some who had enough and to spare.

There was a couple on the island, Tomás Aindrias and his wife Nóra Kearney. They had two daughters, by name Kate and Mary, but Tomás was a poor man. One night he and his wife were together.

'What will we do now?' said the wife. 'We've only a stone of meal left.'

'What will we do, ourselves and the children?' said Tomás.

'Don't worry about that,' said Nora. 'The help of God is nearer than the door. God didn't put a thornbush in the harbour mouth. For he always has a full store if it's His will to scatter with His hand.'

'That's the truth!' said Tomás to Nora. 'You've placed your trust in God; praise be to Him forever!'

'Yes,' said Nora. 'You've finished eating by all appearances.'

'Well,' answered Tomás, 'I've no business to be

124

going to Dingle, as I owe ten pounds to Harrington the shopkeeper already and he wouldn't give me any more credit.'

The next morning early he went to Earraí Beach gathering seaweed. When he went down to the strand he went over to Mary Landers' hole. What was sleeping in the hole but a big seal. He stole up on him holding a big stem of seaweed and he went over to the hole and killed the seal. Then he started to gather the seaweed, but it was very scarce.

'I'll go over to White Island channel' he said to himself.

On his way, what was before him but something better than seaweed, two barrels of flour. He gave high thanks to God; praise be to Him forever!

''Tis true for Nora,' he said to himself. 'The help of God was nearer than the door!'

He didn't worry about the seaweed but about getting the barrels to the top of the cliffs.

Nora was up. 'What's that over there,' she said, 'on your back?'

'Look at it. What did I say last night – that the thornbush was not in the mouth of the harbour. I won't eat a handful of it until I get the second barrel before anyone will be up and about.'

He brought up the second barrel and he ate his breakfast.

''Tis even better than that, Nora,' he said. 'I have killed a fine seal so that we'll have tasty kitchen from the sea. I'll go over and I'll get the seaweed up now.'

He took the donkey with him and there was a fine beach spread out before him. He went down to the rocks at low water so that he could get a pocketful of limpets. What was under the mouth of the rock but a sailor's coat. It was loose but the sleeves were held fast. He didn't want to tear it, and after a while he managed to loosen it. He brought it over to where the seal was and he put it on a rock so that the water would drain from it. He got a grip on the seal and put it up on the back of the donkey. He got the coat nice and dry, and came back to Nora with the fine big seal. He hung out the coat and he got both sides dry. He turned it inside out because the pockets were inside. He opened every one and 'tis how there was a little leather bag in each. There were three hundred yellow sovereigns in one of them and a hundred in another one.

'Now, Nora,' he said, 'praise be to God that we have our fill to eat and drink. I don't need to be doffing my cap looking for credit from Harrington. Now we are able to pay him back our debts. I'll go to Dingle today.'

He and the boat crew set off and arrived in the town.

'Well,' he said to Harrington, 'I suppose I won't be getting anything on credit today.'

'Tomás,' he said, 'it's hard to refuse you. There's ten pounds written down here against you. You've no wealth to be buying anything but I won't send you away empty. What do you want today, Tomás?'

'I need a bag and a half of meal and eight stone of flour.'

'You'll have to go twenty pounds in debt,' said Harrington.

He gave it to him.

'Take out your account book now,' said Tomás. 'Tell me how much there is there now for the ten pounds that was there at first?'

'It's nineteen pounds now,' said Harrington.

'If it is,' said Tomás, 'it won't be any longer!'

He pulled out his purse and counted it out in

yellow gold.

'Look!' said Harrington. 'Woe betide the man that gave you a refusal!'

'You didn't anyway,' said Tomás. 'Luck and blessings on you!'

Back home, Tomás said to Nora his wife: "Lís Connor the poor widow hasn't a scrap of porridge, nor has her two sons. It's to her that I'm giving the half-bag of meal and the eight stone of flour. There's nobody poor on the island except myself and 'Lís. The other five houses that are there are not bad. Every one of them has a milch cow, and if he has, 'tis hungry milk he has, for they wouldn't give me a drop!'

'Lís came looking for a can of water and the well was at Nora's door. She had two rabbits for them. Nora had a fine cake of bread cooked at that time. Nora gave her a piece of bread and a mug of coffee, but she said, 'I'll give them to Seán and Michael. I won't eat them on you.'

Nora compelled her to eat it. She went out to the room. They had three baskets of potatoes. She filled the can with potatoes for 'Lís and gave her half the cake of bread.

'Take it to them and they can eat it,' she said. 'Come again.'

She came again. Nora gave her a plate of meal and two plates of flour. She said then that she would give her plenty.

The crew of the small boat were going over to the mainland to get seed potatoes. Nora went across with them and she went to Kate Boland, the woman with the small shop. Kate had shop bread, so Nora bought a big loaf of the white bread. Her aunt Kate Kearney had food ready for her. She told her how 'Lís and her two lads were hungry. 'God help us!' said the aunt.

'Isn't that a terrible story.' The aunt gave her a couple of stone of meal and a half-stone of flour with it. Her husband Tim came in.

'Isn't that a sad story, Tim, about 'Lís Connor?'

'What's that story?' said Tim.

'That she hasn't a bite to eat, herself and the two lads.'

Tim went to the potato store and he filled half a bag of potatoes. He brought it over to a boat at the landing-place at Faill Chliadh.

'Now, Nora,' he said, 'there's half a sack of potatoes put into the *naomhóg*!'

When she got back to the island she told her daughter Kate to go to 'Lís and to tell her there was a bag of potatoes for her at the Blasket harbour. They brought the donkey with them and took them happily back to the house.

'Lís came up to Nora. 'Nora,' she said, 'who gave the potatoes to me?'

'Young Tim, my aunt's husband. There's meal and flour all mixed up together from my aunt.'

'Praise be God,' she said, 'that everyone's heart isn't thinking evil!'

She gave her half the loaf and 'Lís had gathered up a month's supply or better than that. It was a lucky evening for her, for until Tomás came from town it was the poorest day she ever had. She was very lucky. Tomás took her son Seán into the fishing boat – a twelve-year-old boy counted at that time for a half-man's share in the fishing. He was bringing home the fish, curing it and selling it. Tomás spoke again to 'Lís: 'You now have the grass of a cow. If you give it to me for a while I'll buy a cow so that we'll all be able to have milk out of her. When Seán and Michael will be able to work for themselves, I'll give her to them.'

He cleared the ground where he had the cow. 'Lís was getting as independent as any of them until her son was twenty-five years old. Tomás gave his daughter Kate to be married to Seán and fifty sovereigns with her as a dowry. Tomás had an uncle at Reask and this uncle died. He had grass for four cows on his land and he left the land to Tomás and his daughter Mary. Tomás left the island and gave the grass of his own cow to Kate and Seán. Seán Connor and his wife and little Kate lived fully satisfied with the island from then on.

The sincerity of Méiní's religious faith could not be doubted by anyone who knew her, but she maintained a healthy, good-humoured scepticism about the clergy. Her own experiences with them had been mixed; the censure of herself and Seán Eoghain for running a shebeen has been mentioned. She loved the element of devilment in human nature and appreciated it when a simple man could score off a cleric. The story of Seán O'Sullivan from Coumeenole was related to Mícheál Ó Gaoithín in a longer composite version than what follows, which I recorded on tape in 1962, when Méiní was approximately eighty-six years of age. She told Mike Pheig that Seán's wife was Siobhán Criomhthain, and a man of his name is recorded as living in Coumeenole in 1850.

Seán O'Sullivan was living over by Coumeenole beach and he had a very nice garden of cabbages. People used to be stealing them at night but Seán was a good-living man who held nothing against anyone and he wouldn't like to put a curse on a single soul. He didn't like the idea of giving evidence in court cases and so he set off one Saturday morning and went to the parish of Ferriter to call on the parish priest.

'Well now, Seán,' said the parish priest, 'what brought you this way today?'

'Oh, Father, 'tis my little garden of cabbages that has been robbed every morning after the night. I'm not a man who likes putting curses on people or going to court, and so I've come instead to you so that you can talk to the people who are at Mass tomorrow.'

'Oh, indeed, Seán,' said the priest, 'is it how you'd think I'd be speaking to the people tomorrow about your miserable patch of cabbages. I wouldn't say anything about it. It isn't worth it, to be giving out about such a little thing at all!'

The next Friday night, Seán set out from Coumeenole with a basket, and he didn't stop until he came to the garden where the priest's cabbages were. He filled his basket with them and took them home with him to Coumeenole.

Everything was fine until the Sunday when the priest was saying Mass. When he had finished saying it he spoke out about the bad day's work that was done by the person who had come robbing his garden and had stolen his cabbages.

'If it's done again,' he said, 'I'll read the Cursing Psalms for my garden!'

Seán was listening that Sunday to the priest and his argument.

When everyone had left the chapel, up he goes to the priest.

'Wasn't it a bad thing, Father, that it wasn't any curse you'd say for my cabbages?'

'It isn't a good thing to do any harm to me,' said the priest, 'and it was right for me to speak about it at Mass. Yes, Seán, remember that no cabbages are as important as the priest's cabbages!'

Married as she was to a fisherman, Méiní was not free from the understandable fear which is the constant companion of the families of those who make their living from the sea. The usual superstitions about the sea formed part of her mental make-up. Some of these were more powerful in some localities than in others. For example, in the Dunquin and Blaskets area the word *rua* (red-haired), was not spoken in a boat, and meeting a red-haired person on the way to the boat was considered particularly unlucky and could cause an expedition to be cancelled. The importance of the sea in her life inevitably resulted in its appearance in Méiní's stories, and my final example is of this type. It does not seem to have had a local origin and has an older feel than many of her other tales. The swallowing of persons by sea-monsters, particularly by sea-serpents, is a well-known motif in Irish mythological tradition.

There was a boat crew in County Clare – eight men working her, going out with lines and spinning-hooks. They used to go a little bit out from the place to the fishing-bank. One very fine day they caught ling and cod and they put out the spinner a few times. The boat was getting leaky because the fish was heavy in it.

'Don't put yourselves out. The day is fine and the sea is calm,' said a man called Simon, one of the crew. 'If it is,' said the captain, Thomas O'Meara, 'a person would be drowned on a fine day as well as a day that would be rough.'

'You are right, Thomas,' said Maurice, another one of the crew. They rowed off with them to the harbour and as they were reaching it, a big wave was coming after them. 'Tis how there was a big sea-serpent. The daughter of a lord in County Cork had been swallowed by it when she was on Ballyheigue beach. The head of the girl stuck in the sea-serpent's throat; her legs went away down the serpent's backside. It wasn't able to draw its breath and because of that it was furious.

It followed the boat so fast that it ended up beside it with its feet on the quay. The beach was drying up at the time and the water went away from the serpent so that it wasn't able to go away when the water drained from it.

'Maurice,' said Thomas, 'would you go down to the house and bring back the scythe and the knife with you. We will get rich from the liver which is in it. We'll have a barrel of oil out of it.'

Maurice gave him the scythe and the big knife.

'Pull on its head now!' said Thomas to Éamonn.

Maurice pulled the scythe against the back of its head and he cut the head from the serpent.

'What's to be done now, Thomas?' asked Maurice.

'Pull the big knife down through the middle of its back. That's the place I'd say you should cut it,' said Éamonn.

They cut it open and what was inside but the daughter of the lord. They took her out. She wasn't dead although partly swallowed by the serpent; but she had no clothes on except pieces of thread. They gave her water to drink. Maurice said, 'There's some life back in her again!'

Thomas threw his breeches to her and he took off the drawers that were inside and they pulled them up on the girl to cover up that much of her. Michael took off his shirt and they put it down on her to cover her body.

'Off with you now!' said Thomas to Éamonn, 'and bring back the donkey and cart. Tell Joan to get the bed ready.'

They were all the time giving the water to the princess and greater strength was coming into her breath. Thomas took her home to his own house and they fixed her into Joan's bed.

'For goodness sake!' said Joan, 'where did you get the girl?'

'We got her,' said her husband Thomas, 'in the belly of the sea-serpent.'

'By my word,' she said, 'if you were to put half a glass of poteen into her, perhaps she'd come to herself!' They lifted her up and they poured a porridge-spoon of the poteen down her.

They left her with Joan and they went to their boat and their fish and the sea-serpent. Around one o'clock the girl let out a screech in her sleep.

'You're safe and sound, little girl,' said Joan.

In the evening when the men came home the girl had come back to her senses and she didn't know where she was. It was about six o'clock in the evening when her sense and her mind had come back and she asked Joan where she was.

'You are in Thomas O'Meara's house,' Joan answered.

The lord was searching for his daughter and the story went around that the daughter was drowned. He was in black sorrow. The crew of the boat heard that a lord in Cork had got tidings that his daughter was drowned.

'Would you have any reluctance,' Thomas said to his crew, 'to set off on the road?'

They set off and they didn't stop until they got to Cork. All the nobles were gathered round because of the death of the daughter. Whatever the sorrow that the lord had, he said to his servants to give a drink to the poor tramps that had arrived.

'Thank you, sir,' said Thomas to the lord. 'They are not tramps at all. We are eight fishermen that have rescued your daughter.'

'Do you have her, dead or alive?' said the father.
'She is alive,' said Thomas.

He went to his wife to say that Martha (for that was his daughter's name) was alive.

'Who told you that?' she said. 'It's probably some blackguard that's coming mocking you!'

When Thomas heard what she had said, he answered, 'If she thinks that, you will be able to come to seek her out and see her. Get clothes to put on her. I won't tell you any more until you test the story for yourself.'

Six of the crew stayed in the lord's house while Maurice and Thomas came with the lord to County Clare. The daughter was in a peaceful sleep when her father came to her.

'Would you say now,' said Thomas, 'that it is your daughter?'

'Indeed it is,' said the father.

'Don't wake her out of her sleep,' said Joan, 'until she wakes up of her own accord.'

And that's the way it was. She slipped awake herself.

'Martha, where have you been since?' the father asked.

'I'll tell you tomorrow,' she said. 'I'll tell you everything then.'

Very soon, Maurice, Thomas and the lord returned to Cork. Now the truth was that the six they had left in Cork after them were drunk. When the lord arrived home, his wife asked him: 'What news do you bring?'

'The news is good,' he said. 'Thanks be to God. We will go and get her tomorrow.'

Thomas and Maurice got up the next morning and when they had finished breakfast the lord and his wife, Thomas and Maurice, set off again to County Clare.

The six that had been left in Cork were drunk and were not able to travel out of the house.

'I'll leave them there,' said the lord, 'until they come to their senses!'

In the morning, Martha was up with her clothes on when her father and mother came. Her mother kissed her with all her heart. In one hour, Thomas told how they got her in the belly of the sea-serpent. She said that it was certainly like what he had said, and that the serpent was not able to breathe and so had swallowed her.

Thomas took the father down to the harbour, and the serpent was lying there.

'That's the serpent now!' said Thomas.

The lord made powerful men of the eight that were in the boat.

'If any misfortune grips you from now on, I will settle every problem and hardship that will come your way,' said the lord.

He took his daughter back to Cork, and by that time the six men had come to their senses. The daughter took the chains off their hands, and the Lord sent the six of them back to County Clare. The lord's daughter didn't do any more swimming again until the day of her death.

14

THE LATER MARRIED YEARS

Robin Flower was well acquainted with Méiní and Seán Eoghain and some of her stories in the collection of the Folklore Commission were recorded by him. On the occasion of Gobnait Kennedy's telling of the story of Purty Deas Squarey, he writes that 'Méiní lit a candle at my elbow to throw light on my book, and setting my chair against Gobnait and resting the book on the table, I prepared to follow her voice with flying pencil.'

By this time, Gobnait Kennedy had been a close friend of Méiní for at least ten years. Tomás Ó Criomhthain records how he and Gobnait's father Dan Kennedy together built the little house for 'Bell' high in the Upper Village; it may well be that as a girl Gobnait had come to the Blaskets with her father and was familiar with its people. On February 4, 1911, in Ballyferriter, she married Pats Shéamuis Guiheen, the son of Paddy Shéamuis (who is misleadingly referred to as Pats Hamish in English translations of *An tOileánach*) and of Kate Ní Chriomhthain, Tomás's sister. Pats and Gobnait lived in the Lower Village and their house stood with its back to Méiní's house, about fifty yards to the south-east. Pats was a regular visitor to Seán Eoghain, and it was natural for their wives to form a close friendship, especially

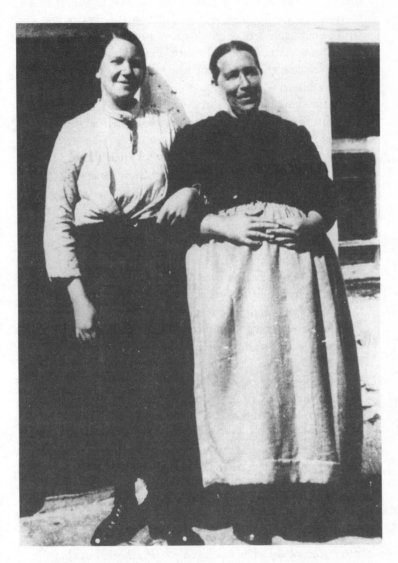

(Left to right) *Gobnait Kennedy, a fine storyteller and wife to Pats Shéamuis Ó Guithín, with Méiní in middle age*

so since they were both blow-ins from the mainland. Gobnait had brought on to the island her sister Méin who was reputed to be a bit simple. She was well-known to the islanders, who called her 'Méin of the Weaver' because of her father's occupation. After Gobnait's death, Pats did his best to look after Méin on the island but was eventually forced to put her in a home.

In the same month, February 1911, Méiní's grandfather, old Seán Keating, died in Dunquin. News reached the island that he was failing and Méiní came out to be with her grandmother Méireas and her mother. When she had been there two days the old man died and Méiní was chosen to go with the men to get the material for the wake, the presence of a woman being obligatory on such occasions. There were, according to her account, two barrels of porter, white bread, tea, tobacco and clay pipes, so that, in her words, 'Seán Keating was buried in the blessed graveyard with as much decency as anybody that ever went there.' She remarks that the Dunquin people had treated him, who had come among them as a boy, exactly as one of themselves, so that he never thought of returning to his father's and mother's relations whom he had left behind him at St Michael's Well in Ballinskelligs.

It is not easy to gauge the extent to which the Great War affected the lives of the islanders. Potatoes and fish would have been as plentiful as ever, although supplies of meal for making bread may at times have been short. Certainly, the tradition among the older islanders was that times were hard, but in August 1916 a dramatic upturn in their fortunes took place. On the twenty-third of that month, the British cargo ship *Quebra* was wrecked on the Lóchar rock on the west of the island while on a voyage from New York to Liverpool. Initial reports by the Lloyd's agent at Ventry suggested that thirty-four of the crew managed to get ashore, but that the captain and two sailors were missing. The *Quebra* was a vessel with a displacement of 4538 tons and had been built only four years before by W. Grey and Co, for the Mercantile Steamship line. At the time of the shipwreck, she was carrying a general cargo and large quantities of this floated ashore or were taken from the wreck by local fishermen.

Although he wrongly dates the wreck of the *Quebra* as happening in May, Maurice O'Sullivan gives an account which accords well with the recollections of their elders' accounts given by the surviving Blasket islanders. The first Maurice knew of the accident was when, from his school desk, he saw the King and the *Poncán* hurrying down to the harbour carrying their thole-pins and ropes. Very soon, the inhabitants of the island, almost to a man, were gathered above the spit of Seals' Cove near Shingle Strand (Tráigh Earraí), which was covered in wreckage of all kinds. Every *naomhóg* on the island was busy collecting the boxes and barrels floating on the water. The young boy remembered particularly the crates of apples and boxes of chocolates that were carried up to the houses.

At this point only the two masts and the funnel of the ship were visible above the waterline. Three boats had set off from the vessel as she foundered, according to the captain's account, and in two of these the bulk of the crew got to safety in Dingle Bay. The third contained the Captain, the mate, and one injured sailor. Escorted by a *naomhóg*, this third boat was able to reach the island harbour, the injured man being taken to Micil Nell's house. Máire Guiheen, who was a child of about seven at the time, remembered hearing that the captain soon fell asleep exhausted at the house of Maurice Keane (Maras Mhuiris), who was in his middle forties at the time and active in salvaging the cargo with his crew. His daughter Kate was particularly struck by the gold ring on the captain's finger and told her friend Máire Guiheen about it.

Tomás Ó Criomhthain was one of the few islandmen

not to be able to collect his share of the wreckage. The only person he had with him at the time was his elderly brother and nobody invited him to share in crewing a boat. He recalls that the captain said that the *Quebra* had everything that feeds mankind except drink, this last circumstance no doubt preventing the development of a *Whisky Galore!* situation.

A plentiful supply of bacon floated ashore and it was possible to salvage some of the flour because, according to Seán Ó Guithín, the middle section of the barrels remained dry under a damp outer skin. No sugar was salvaged, to the disappointment of the islanders, as it dissolved in the seawater.

Maurice O'Sullivan recounts how he and his pal Tomás O'Connor, returning from viewing the wreck, saw two men, one of whom was Pats Léan Ó Guithín, examining a decorated box full of watches in a cave. They were quickly chased away. According to Pats's nephew, three boxes of watches were recovered, and Maurice O'Sullivan says that after the shipwreck every man, woman and child had a watch in their pocket, though whether or not they were in working condition after their immersion is unknown. Máire Guiheen records particularly the fate of a fine tea-set which was salvaged. A cup from the set was later given as a love-token to her sister Eileen by Seán O'Shea, who was drowned some years later.

Among the clothes recovered were women's stockings, boxes of shirts, cloth caps, raincoats and rubber overshoes. The cargo was important to the islanders not only because of what they could salvage for their own use but because much of it was saleable on the mainland. Ó Criomhthain says that hundreds of pounds were made by the islanders in this way.

Particularly vivid in the memory of the islanders was the amount of leather in bundles which they were able to recover. Seán Ó Guithín says that as a result of this a shoemaker called O'Sullivan from the mainland stayed for a while at the house of Maurice O'Sullivan's father at *Tigh na Leacan*. Seán added that, thirty years after the wreck, he and Seán Kearney (Seán Sheásaí) found leather at Seals' Cove, one and a quarter miles north-east of the site of the wreck.

No less than for the rest of the islanders, the wreck of the *Quebra* proved a godsend for Méiní and her family. Her husband was still active as a fisherman and her son Séamus was in his late teens and well able to lend a hand, so there was no trouble manning their *naomhóg* to garner their share of the wreckage and cargo. Méiní's account to Mike Pheig Sayers contains some nice touches:

I had never any lack of anything from the day the Church bound us together. But that would not count for everything. Sadness used to come too. 'Twas how one year would be good for us and another would go against us on the island. I tell you we had call for pride for we always could bring something in the hand to the mouth. I'll always remember the year the boat went aground on Carraig a' Lóchair – we really needed that boat to be wrecked that time, because the war was heavy on us and food was cut off. I heard the crash the vessel made about nine o'clock at night. I didn't remember anything but a nice calm night. 'Twas little that we were expecting that it was a vessel that had run aground on such a night without a breath of wind or rain. About eight o'clock next morning I was out herding cows when Martin Kearney met me from the west looking pale as if he had seen something which had shaken him:

'What's wrong, Martin Tom?'

'There's a big vessel after going aground on the north side of the island on Carraig a' Lóchair.'

I'm not like Mary Doody who knew every rock

above and below the water from the Black Head to the Gob (a promontory near the village). I was as blind as I ever was as to where Carraig a' Lóchair was.

When you looked out on the wreck you wouldn't see anything on the sea but wreckage and wood and chests and barrels and cotton. We got hold of our share of the cargo as well as everyone else. It gave us plenty and we didn't feel the war years or the shortages which followed them, but we had flour and meat and fat stranded on the beach for us. The island people gathered as much as they could of everything so that it wasn't the Island of Hunger in those years, but the Island of Plenty.

15

BIRTHS, MARRIAGES – AND BOOKS

Two events worthy of note occurred in Méiní's circle during 1917. Her stepson Eoghan was married in February to Bridget Flaherty, from Clogher, between Dunquin and Ballyferriter. Bridget's sister Joanie (Joanie Bhán) was married to Tomás Dunleavy, known as 'Bell', whom she had met in America. Unfortunately, Bridget died a few years after her marriage, which was childless. Eoghan eventually moved to a little house at the top of the island village, and in old age he settled on the mainland at Ballinaraha. It was also in 1917 that Méiní's grandmother, Méireas, died in Dunquin. In contrast to her full account of her grandfather's death, Méiní gives no description of her grandmother's death or burial.

In the same year in April arrived Brian Ó Ceallaigh. He was an enigmatic character, a Kerryman who had won Irish prizes at TCD and eventually died in Yugoslavia. On both his visits (he returned in 1918) he played a key part in the island story by sensing Ó Criomhthain's literary potential and encouraging him to write *Allagar na hInise* (*Island Cross-Talk*) and later *An tOileánach* on which his fame rests. Méiní knew of Ó Ceallaigh's visit but spoke little about him. He brought balls for the boys of the island and the girls got sweets. These were, no doubt, enjoyed by Méiní's children, of whom the younger, Máire, was only fifteen at the time.

The island was not immune from the flu epidemic which passed across Europe in 1918 in the wake of the war. Father Mac Craith was curate in Ballyferriter at this time, and he rode around on a saddlehorse. He was known for being as good a doctor as a priest and during that time of illness and loss his ministrations on the island were greatly valued, especially by such as Méiní who had a natural interest in the care of the sick.

Late in November 1918 the sea-captain known as 'Hix' arrived at the island with the news that the Great War was over. Méiní brought the news to Seán Eoghain, who, with his customary boisterous cynicism retorted: 'May the Devil take him from me, the biggest liar on the coast of Kerry, or of Ireland itself!'

Early in 1919 news of a possible match for Seán Keane, son of the island king, Pats Mhicí, came from Dingle. The prospective swain gathered up two of his pals to accompany him to the town to bring matters a stage further on. The first of these supporters was Pats Mhuiris Keane (known as the 'Leehuck') and the other a Daly boy, most likely Paddy Mharas, whose sister Neans was married to Pats Mhuiris. The next day, Seán Eoghain returned from a visit to the neighbours and was met by Méiní, eager to get news of the success or failure of the much-heralded expedition. The abrasive Seán Eoghain attacked her for her inquisitiveness, taking a verbal swipe at Seán Keane for going outside the island for his bride.

'Did you never hear tell,' said Méiní, 'that far-off cows have long horns?' Seán Eoghain retorted by criticising the accuracy of Méiní's rendering of the old saying. It was always his custom to have the last word on any topic.

One or two mornings afterwards, Tomás Ó Criomhthain came across to Méiní to tell her that the King was setting off to the mainland for his son's wedding. She had difficulty in waking up her son Séamus who was to accompany the bridegroom with two other men and three women. When Maurice, Méiní's stepson, who was still a bachelor, returned from a poor day's fishing, in which dogfish constituted his only catch, he heard that the initial wedding-party had left and that he was to follow the next day with the rest of the guests.

The bride who returned with Seán Keane was known on the island as 'Mag an Rí', being the King's daughter-in-law. Although their married life was to be relatively short, Seán dying of blood-poisoning in early 1934, they had a family of seven. It is likely that all these children were delivered by Méiní. The youngest child was the baby girl born in 1933 after Méiní had left the island, for whose birth she was called back to act as midwife. This was almost certainly the last occasion on which she returned.

Around about 1920, so Tomás relates, Seán Eoghain built a new room on to the house, with a felt roof. This was occupied by Séamus, now twenty-three, and his step-brother Maurice, who was to be married the following year – indeed it may have been built in anticipation of this situation. The two young men were frightened by inexplicable noises which came from the roof at odd times, and were on the point of abandoning the room on the assumption that they were being visited by evil spirits. Tomás himself claimed to have resolved the problem, as, digging in his potato field nearby, he noticed a big black crow on the roof of the room being attacked by a dog which jumped up to get at it. The origin of the evil spirits was thus explained and the room came back into favour.

The next important event in the life of Seán Eoghain's household was the marriage of his son Maurice to Kate Manning on 5 February 1921, when he was thirty-one years of age. Kate had come from her home in Kilvickadownig in

Ventry Parish to be assistant teacher in the island school in September 1907, and would have known Maurice for the thirteen years before they married. Máire Guiheen in *An tOileán a Bhí* describes him as a lovely strong man and a good musician. The couple stayed fourteen years on the island after their marriage, eventually leaving in 1935 when Kate took up a post in Murreagh. During ten or eleven of these years the couple seem to have shared the house with Méiní and Seán Eoghain and became the parents of a daughter and a son. The conditions must have been extremely cramped, especially in the years before Méiní's own children left for America; it is said that relations were often strained between Méiní and her stepdaughter-in-law. This in turn may have had some part to play in Méiní's comparatively rapid departure from the island after Seán Eoghain's death, especially as by that time the elder stepson had been widowed and he had returned to live temporarily in the family home. Eibhlís O'Sullivan, referring in her letter to George Chambers to the death of Seán Eoghain, implies that Méiní was no longer considered as having any rights in the house.

Robin Flower in his description of the household while Kate's daughter was a baby nowhere suggests any such friction but he depicts the daughter-in-law as teasing the old man for his own love of white bread and sugar. He had been calling down curses on them for their effect on the health of the island children.

In 1921 died Michael Keane, otherwise known as 'Mikil Chuainí' or just 'Cuainí'. He was the son of the sea-captain Maurice Keane (known as Muiris na Tinte) who had been born on Inishtooskert. Cuainí apparently owed his nickname to the fact that his mother was Mary Counihan from Ballinvoher near Annascaul. His wife Nell Guiheen was always referred to as Nell Chuainí. Their son Pádraig, known as 'Casht' was a gifted musician who passed on his talents to his son Seán and his family. Cuainí had a brother Seán (known as 'Balt') who was married to Méiní's sister Junie. Even without such a family connection, it would have been inevitable that Seán Eoghain, as an island character, would have been invited to Cuainí's wake. The entertainment, as he recounted to Tomás, included a whole barrel of porter. Returning to his own house late at night, and settling down to take a rest before returning to the wake, he found his house invaded by eight men who sat down to a meal. As they were leaving, another group from the mainland arrived and Méiní had to prepare a meal for them also.

Around the year 1926, Méiní's daughter Máire decided she would leave the island for America where she had many relations in the Springfield area. Her mother was shattered by this decision but she was sensible enough to know that such a move was all but inevitable. Her husband was growing old, she herself was only fifty and her long widowhood would bring unavoidable loneliness. This would be intensified if her son Séamus were also to decide to leave, as so many of his contemporaries had done. She explained movingly to Mike Pheig her sorrow at her daughter's departure. 'That was the first time,' she said, 'that the island became dark around me.'

Máire promised her that she would return every four years to see her, and although this was impossible in the years of the Second World War, she faithfully kept the spirit, if not strictly the letter, of her promise, particularly so in Méiní's extreme old age. This kept up the old woman's spirits, although the partings were painful.

Séamus, as Méiní had feared, soon decided to follow his sister, but he found it impossible, as a result of his erratic schooling, to satisfy the educational requirements for immigrants into the United States, and had to settle instead for Canada, where the entry requirements were less strict. Some men from his own area, including his almost exact contemporary, Séamus 'Twoee' Kavanagh from Gleann Luic, had gone from time to time to Canada, but Kerry people were not as plentiful as in the Boston area and Séamus found it impossible to settle. Shortly after his father's death he returned to the island and kept close contact with his mother until his own sudden death at age sixty-six. Even when he eventually settled on the mainland he spent a great deal of time in fishing around the islands, and lived 'inside' for long spells, long after his mother had left.

During his final years, Seán Eoghain became increasingly infirm and housebound and greatly missed Máire and Séamus. Before he died, Máire had married an Irishman, Austin Kilcoyne, and had begun her family. Méiní told Mike Pheig how his mother Peig Sayers used to come and sit beside Seán Eoghain's bed and read him the letters which came from Máire, a situation which Máire must easily have imagined. Peig said that she did this because Seán Eoghain had looked after her in her own day of hardship. In one of these letters Máire announced the birth of her son.

In 1928, Tomás Ó Criomhthain's island diary *Allagar na hInise* was published, followed in 1929 by his classic tale of island life *An tOileánach*. Although the second book was widely translated and eventually received the accolade of publication in English in Penguin Books, there was naturally a certain amount of jealousy on the island and some partly justified resentment at his interpretation of certain aspects of its life. The main point of dispute seems to have been Tomás's insistence that his father had helped many people on the island, a claim which was held to proceed entirely from his own imagination and to reflect on the capacities of the other islanders. Shortly after the contents of the book became known on the island, and its defects had been emphasised by a tincture of begrudgery, we get a glimpse of the old abrasive Seán Eoghain as he talks angrily about Tomás, who had been his sparring partner in so many arguments. Kruger Kavanagh, who visited Seán Eoghain after the book had been published, told me in the early 1950s (recorded by me then), that he remembered the old man saying: 'I'd prefer to be chewing manure in my mouth than listening to the red lies told by that little scrap of a man.' Truly a case of a prophet without honour.

16

SLÁN LE SEÁN EOGHAIN

During the Great War and right up to the 1930s it was the custom of the Dunquin lads to row over to the island on calm Sunday afternoons for dancing. The prominent musicians at the time were Pádraig Daly ('Paddy Mharas') and Pádraig Keane ('Casht'). The Séamus 'Twoee' Kavanagh already referred to, and who died at an advanced age in 1991, was one of those who made such regular expeditions prior to his departure for Canada in 1930. He himself generally crewed a *naomhóg* along with Seán Moriarty (Seán 'Tull'), a neighbour from Gleann Luic and Pádraig de Brún (*'An Pápa'*). Another *naomhóg* was frequently manned by Seán Keane ('Balt'), Méiní's brother-in-law, accompanied by one of his sons and frequently by Tomás Guiheen ('Plate') who, as has been noted, had been Seán Eoghain's best man in 1896. Méiní's house, so easily accessible to the harbour, would have been at this time an obvious port of call for these mainlanders.

Throughout all these years, Méiní had to work harder than ever before. While Kate Manning was at school she would have had to take charge of the children, and as Seán Eoghain grew more infirm many of the heavy jobs such as drawing seaweed to manure the potato-patch fell to her. In the winter evenings, in common with the other island women, she knit socks and jerseys for her men-folk from the coarse hard wool which was still being spun by the older women on the island. The island weaver, Eoghan Bán O'Connor, was dead and his loom no longer in use; Méiní's own grandfather had not been weaving for some years prior to his death in 1911. Dan Kennedy brought over cloth for sale to the islanders and these were fashioned into garments by tailors such as Máire Scanlon's father.

As the 1930s began, the flames of Seán Eoghain's fiery, combative spirit were burning low. Although the two sons of his first marriage were still with him, he pined for the children of his middle age and the letters that Peig read to him were but a feeble consolation, even when one of them brought news of a second son for Máire and Austin in Springfield. As Méiní said, 'There was nothing now in the bed but a skeleton paying no attention to what was going on.'

During the first days of 1932, Méiní's neighbour 'Lís O'Sullivan wrote to her friend George Chambers telling him that Seán Eoghain was seriously ill. Jerry O'Shea, the father-in-law of Pats Tom Kearney had died only a few days before, and the island people, affected by the closeness of death, were reluctant to go out of doors in the dark except in a group, since thoughts of death were still mingled with those of the fairy world. 'Everyone is frightened,' Lís reported, 'until the dead person is buried a month or so.'

Two months later on 4 March 1932 at two in the morning Seán Eoghain breathed his last. Thirty years later, Méiní poured out her feelings on that occasion to Mike Pheig Sayers:

> I was left on my own, an old old woman without strength in my leg, without a tooth in my head, without happiness in store for me, waiting for the glorious messenger to come and call me.

Her emphasis on her old age was exaggerated, since she was as yet only in her middle fifties, but her grief was certainly genuine, as was her assessment of the general difficulty of her position. Her children were gone from her as well as her husband, and she knew in her heart that she had also lost her home, now that there were no men living there but her stepsons, Eoghan a widower, and Maurice with his wife and family.

Thanks to 'Lís O'Sullivan we can follow closely the sequence of events immediately after Seán Eoghain's death. She tells how the eldest son and his wife and two more lads went out in the *naomhóg* to get the material for the wake (in fact it must have been the second son as Eoghan was already a widower). By long-standing tradition it was considered essential that a woman should go on this expedition. If none could be got to leave the island, a female friend or relative was picked up in Dunquin on the way to Dingle.

A motor-car was hired in Dunquin which made its way over the Clasach pass to Ventry and Dingle, while the two boys who had come in the *naomhóg* set off north to Ballyferriter to ask the priest to come to Dunquin the next day. In Dingle, a motor-lorry was hired which brought the coffin, a half-barrel of porter, white bread, jam and a few bottles of whiskey. The supplies reached the island in the early evening about sixteen hours after the death. As the coffin was carried past the beehive storehouse called the *Púicín Buí* into the house, the old women began the *olagón*, the cry of mourning, which would break out at recognised intervals as the evening passed towards the dawn. The dead man was dressed in his new suit and all the islanders came to view the corpse and to say a prayer for his soul. The old people touched his cold hand, an act which was believed to take away the danger of being haunted by the dead man, but the young children were too scared even to do that.

Two *naomhóga* came in from the mainland so that their

crews could join the wake. Men like 'Plate' would certainly have been there, along with 'Balt', who was married to Méiní's sister Junie, and one or two of their sons. At times the mourners gathered around the corpse, when prayers were said and keening was heard. At other times the company would gather around the fire in the big room, more relaxed in mood. Stories were swopped, and as 'Lís O'Sullivan wrote, 'We spent the night happily.' 'Lís also remarks how lonely Méiní seemed that night, longing for her own son and daughter to be there with her in her sorrow.

By this time some of the old traditions were beginning to break down, even in the Blaskets, and we do not know whether, for example, *punann na marbh*, the sheaf of straw for the dead, was placed beside the corpse so that those praying could kneel upon it. It is certain that as midnight approached the Rosary was recited. Méiní herself had a strong sense of the dramatic, and as dawn broke her voice would have been heard reciting the lament for the soul as it left the body:

The cock is crowing and the dawn is breaking,
And my love, he himself, going home away from me.

By eight o'clock, those who were not going to cross to Dunquin for the burial were beginning to drift away to their houses and some badly needed sleep.

That Saturday morning the procession of *naomhóga* left the island at half-past nine. A storm was blowing up and they thought it better to be going early before it got any worse. The canoe which carried the coffin was accompanied by five others in line astern. No sooner did they arrive at Dunquin pier than the wind arose, making it impossible for the islanders to return that day. They were used to that situation and all of them would have relatives and friends on the mainland with whom they could bed down for the night, after, one assumes, a convivial evening.

The coffin was carried up the cruelly steep slope which led from the pier to the top of the cliff, and then the cortège made its way down through Ballykeen and Ballinaraha to the cross near the creamery where the road branched off to the little graveyard in Baile an Teampaill, across the stream from Ballinahow. Here Seán Eoghain was laid to rest almost in the shadow of the church which Father Mangan had built in 1857, around about the time when Seán Eoghain himself was born. Méiní was now at another crossroads in her life.

17

WIDOWHOOD

When she had passed through the initial stages of her mourning for her husband, Méiní began to come to terms with the position in which she found herself. Although there is some reason to believe that she did not always get on well with her stepdaughter-in-law Kate Manning – and living together in such cramped quarters it would have been strange indeed if there was not occasional friction between the two housewives – it cannot be said that she was in any sense forced out of the house against her will. Having married a man so much older than herself, she may well have considered it fitting that control of the home should pass to her stepsons on his death. That this would appear the natural sequence of events was reinforced by the double consideration that her own children were across the Atlantic and that her mother Máire Keating was alive in Dunquin, being cared for by her grandson 'Billy' (Maurice) Keane.

According to her own account to Mike Pheig Sayers, Méiní made up her mind about six months after her husband's death to leave the island. There is no reason to doubt the substantial accuracy of her recollection on this point and September 1932, when the nights were drawing in and the equinoctial gales were expected, appears a likely date. We know that she was certainly off the island by the summer of 1933 when a daughter was born to Mag an Rí. Méiní's return to the island to assist at this birth was unusual enough to be recollected locally.

When Méiní decided to bring to an end her island stay of thirty-six years she prepared to move to her mother's house in Ballykeen the few belongings that could be said to belong to her. The obvious person to assist her was the Seán Keane we have mentioned. He had taken over as island postman from his father, the late King, and was continuing the twice-weekly journeys, when weather permitted, to collect the post on the mainland. On the occasion of Méiní's exodus he was assisted by Seán Pheats Tom Ó Ceárnaigh, then a boy of nineteen, who told me that he particularly remembers Méiní bringing across her own mattress.

There on the cliff to greet her on her arrival – or so she tells us – was her school friend Kate Moriarty. She had been her bridesmaid for the elopement so many long years before, and although the two women had met many times in the intervening years, there were long periods during which they had seen little or nothing of each other. Méiní spoke warmly of Kate, remarking how deeply she appreciated the renewal of their friendship and the many clay pipes of tobacco they were to smoke together as they gossiped about their girlhood escapades, especially their flirtations as teenagers with the Blasket men. It may cause some surprise in our day to reflect that Méiní's use of tobacco, which continued to the end of her days, originated as a cure, recommended by a doctor, for a suspected heart condition.

The home to which Méiní returned retained many of the features of that which she had left, for material changes came slowly in that society. Her grandfather, the weaver, and her grandmother were long since on the 'way of truth' and her mother Máire Keating was largely bedridden. After her grandfather's death and before Méiní's return, her sister

Junie, who had a large family, sent her son Billy to live in the house with Máire, and in spite of her infirmity she was enabled with his help to carry on as agent of Willie Long, the Ballyferriter merchant, and his son-in-law Pats. She supplied flour and meal, and the islanders continued to call at her home for their requirements.

In spite of her married name of Dunlevy, and her maiden name of O'Shea, Méiní continued, like her mother, to be called by her grandfather's name of Keating. It was relatively common for persons in that area to inherit nicknames or patronymics from grandparents. Because she was thus known by her grandfather's name, there has been some confusion in local recollection between Méiní and her mother.

After her husband's death, Méiní became eligible, though relatively young, for the state widow's pension, which was her sole source of income until she received the old age pension. Her wants were few, and, as in the case of the majority of the local people, there were many gifts of money, clothing and special food from their relatives in the United States, particularly from those in the Boston and Springfield areas.

Ballykeen was busy at this time as, shortly after Méiní's return, a new two-storey house was begun in 1934 by the Sheehy family, who were moving out of the smaller house beside the old coastguard's shelter. Old Máire Keating, though by this time on her deathbed, was still in full possession of her senses. Visited one day by her grandson Billy, she told him that if she died he was to keep the fact a secret from the workmen building Sheehy's house, as the tradition was that at the announcement of a death all work would cease in the area. That very evening, she died.

Méiní was grievously stricken by her mother's death; she said she would have preferred anything to the empty chair. She took solace in visiting other elderly women in Dunquin, among them Máire Sheehy, Kateen Sheehy and Máire

Russell. The last-named, who was married to John Long, lived at the *tobar* up on the Clasach road leading directly between Eagle Mountain and Croaghmarhin to Ventry. She was about seventy-six at the time of Méiní's return to Dunquin, and had established a reputation as a fine storyteller, some of whose tales have been recorded. Her sister Kate was a near neighbour of Méiní, living with her husband at the Muileann just above where the Dunquin river enters the sea.

Méiní's loneliness was lightened also by the large number of her relatives living around her in Dunquin. Her sister Junie lived just down the laneway from the old weaver's house, and she and her husband 'Balt' had nine children. At the time of her mother's death Méiní's son Séamus decided to leave Canada and to return to West Kerry. From time to time he lived with his mother but was more often fishing from the Blaskets with his stepbrothers Eoghan and Maurice.

In this same year as her mother's death, Méiní's nephew Billy Keane, together with his friend 'Tull' Moriarty, began to build a house into which Méiní was soon to move. Beside the weaver's house was the remains of an old chapel-of-ease which had been abandoned at the time of the building of the new church in Ballintemple, Dunquin. We read of its last being used as residence of Father Brasbie whose provocatively trumpeted conversion to Protestantism in 1844 has been mentioned. The house that Billy and Seán built was on the site of this old 'Keating chapel', and some of its stones were used in its construction. This last act was reputed to have brought ill-luck to the builders: Billy Keane later developed some form of poisoning which was described as gangrene but did not prove fatal. The old weaver's house, from which Méiní moved at around this time, was allowed to fall into its present state of ruin and in course of time the new house began to be looked on as Méiní's own.

Méiní's work as a midwife was, needless to say, well

known in Dunquin and she continued to help out with mainland births from time to time. Round about this time she began to work as a childminder and domestic for Dan Lynch, a teacher in Burnham, Dingle, who lived at Dunquin with his wife, a daughter of the merchant Willie Long. Each morning she crossed the Red Glen to her work. There were four children in the Lynch family, Méiní's chief responsibility, and here no doubt her nursing skills were frequently called upon. The Lynches usually kept a cow and a calf, and Mike Mistéal from Ballinahow who worked there in his late teens remembers Méiní milking each day. As Mike remarks, Méiní had a better knowledge of cattle than many a farmer at that time. When the cow calved, for instance, she suggested that some milk should be left in the udder to prevent milk fever. She was as good a midwife for a cow as for a woman. Dressed in her black skirt, with her shawl around her shoulders, she would do the housework and cook the meals, pausing from time to time to take a few pulls from her beloved *dúidín*.

In the vicinity lived Seán Dinny Garvey, originally from Carhoo above Dunquin, who had spent a number of years in the United States. After his return to his native place he lived in a variety of houses, but at this time, up into the 1940s he was living with the Ó Luing family of Baile an Ghleanna, and gloried in the nickname of 'The Yarker'. He used to meet Méiní on her way to and from Dan Lynch's house, calling her, for some unknown reason 'Robin of the South'. It is said that he had a soft spot for her but by this time she was in her sixties and even if he had got around to proposing marriage, it is very doubtful if she would have given it a second thought.

In the middle 1940s, Mrs Máirín Sheehy (Máirín Daly) had to spend two years on an orthopaedic frame because of a spinal complaint. Every single day during that time, Méiní came to visit her. They would play cards together, and Méiní kept Máirín's spirits up during her long ordeal by talking to her about the Blaskets and by treating her to recitals of her considerable stock of folktales and stories. When Méiní herself lay grievously ill at the end of her life, Máirín was able to help her family in looking after her and keeping up her spirits as she herself had done for Máirín twenty years before.

In her own right Méiní was still a noteworthy person among islanders and Dunquin people alike and she did her part in keeping up the old traditions. Dr Joe Daly believed that Méiní was the last woman in the Dunquin district to keep up the practice of the *olagón* lament; he himself had heard her. There was no question of payment, at least in this district, for this service of lamentation – it came from the heart of women who had known terrible loss and sorrow. Immediately after a death, there was no keening or lamentation. Tears were shed in silence until the corpse was laid out for the wake. If there was a clock, it was stopped at the time of death to signify that for the dead person time was no more.

We must not imagine that when she left the island Méiní lost contact with the island people. In fact she was able to keep much closer links with the Blasket people than she had been able to maintain with her own mainland relatives during the thirty-five years she spent 'inside'. Apart from a few fishermen and a handful of professional people, there was no need for mainlanders to cross the frequently rough Blasket Sound. For the islanders, on the other hand, contact with the mainland was an economic and social necessity. The days when the island people had been self-sufficient were long since over; they increasingly needed flour, sugar, tea, tobacco and lighting oil as their standard of living began to approximate to that of their mainland cousins. In fine weather, the able-bodied, particularly among the island men, made their way to Sunday Mass in Dunquin and were welcomed and hospitably treated by their mainland relatives. Méiní's son, Séamus, who spent a great deal of his time living on and fishing from the Blaskets, provided a special link and source of information as to what was going on in the life of the island. The sons of her sister Junie, who cared for her in Séamus's absences, were themselves involved in fishing contacts with it.

As the years passed and life on the island became comparatively harder, the tendency to marry on to the mainland grew more pronounced. The King of the island himself, Pats Mhicí Keane, was married to a Dunquin woman from Carhoo (Ferriter's Quarter), and as early as 1918 his daughter Cáit, the Princess, married John Casey, who lived beside the church. She was an important focus of attention for visiting islanders. 'Lís O'Sullivan, in her letters to George Chambers, has artlessly but movingly chronicled this growing tendency to settle on the mainland. She herself, who was married to Tomás Ó Criomhthain's son Seán, moved out in 1942, though not to Dunquin. At about the same time, Peig Sayers, the doyenne of the island storytellers had moved with her son and brother-in-law to Baile Bhiocáire, where her childhood home had stood. In 1947, the Princess's niece, Máire Guiheen, moved to the mainland on her marriage to Labhrás Ó Ciobháin of Ballinaraha, which was within easy walking distance of Méiní's house.

The final exodus from the island was rapidly approaching, though since many of the islanders kept some sort of a shelter on the island for the fishing season one cannot specify accurately the final dates of leaving. By November 1953, when the official evacuation took place, a high proportion of those who left had settled with their old people in the Dunquin area, partly to keep the link with the fishing grounds they knew, but also possibly out of a natural feeling that made them want to keep touch, if only by sight, with what had been their home. By congregating in one place they could maintain the links of friendship formed on the island and keep the *naomhóg* crews intact. Seán 'Casht' Keane and his wife Bríd were among the first of the main body to move, bringing with them their first child Gearóid, the last youngster of the island. They settled in Ballinahow in a house vacated by Ulick Moran, who had moved up to the midlands under a government scheme of Irish-speaking resettlement. This scheme was also responsible for the departure of a Kavanagh family from Ballinaraha and of the O'Connors from the same townland who were the last Protestant family in the area. Both these homesteads were replaced by Blasket people, the first by Pat Mitchell ('The Fiagach'), Eoghan Dunlevy, (Méiní's stepson), and her own son Séamus. The O'Connors were replaced by Seán Pheats Tom Ó Ceárnaigh and his wife 'Lís 'Line' Guiheen; another islander. 'Lís's brother Mike had also moved to Dunquin. In the newly-built cottages were living old Maurice Mhuiris Keane and his family, Maurice Daly ('Dawley') and his wife, Seán Mhike Léan Guiheen and his brother Maurice, Maurice Daly's brothers Tom and Patrick, and Seáinín Mhicil O'Sullivan with his brothers.

Méiní was considerably older than most of the people who settled down in Dunquin from the island. The elderly parents they brought with them would have more in common with her, though opportunities for meeting would have been more limited than on the island. Nevertheless, as her eighties approached, the young islanders who lived near her, and who had contact with her through her son and her nephews, helped to keep up her morale.

In those years there was a further source of pleasure as her daughter Máire Kilcoyne began to make again the regular visits which the Second World War had made impossible. Although the partings at the end of these visits were painful, the visits kept her spirits up, and Máire was able to provide comforts and care for her mother which her local relatives had not been in a position to do. Máire brought news of her own family to their grandmother and the photographs and stories she brought got eager attention. One thing, however, Máire was not able to do. She could not persuade her mother to move into surroundings more comfortable than the bare little cottage on the cliffside. To it she clung on, virtually to the end of her days.

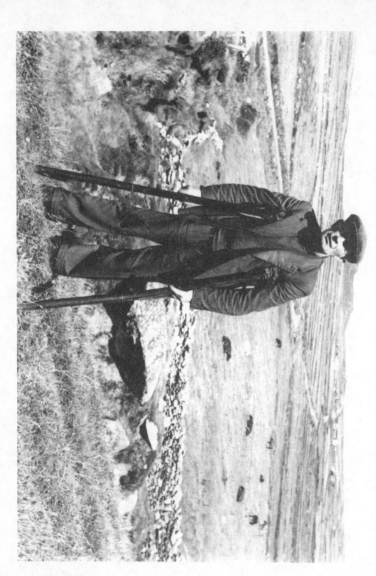

Martin Keane, Méiní's nephew, at Béal Átha. The site of the new Blasket Centre is to the left.

18

THE TWILIGHT AND THE DARK

I first met Martin Keane, Méiní's nephew, in December 1954 and we became firm friends for the remaining eleven years of his life. At that time he was living with his brother at the Muileann, just above where the Dunquin river enters the sea at Béal Átha. Along with his brothers Billy (Maurice) and Bobby (Thomas) he made himself responsible for Méiní who was now approaching her eightieth year. Martin, who was crippled and got around only on crutches, could not do any fishing which involved long journeys, though he was able to look after some lobster-pots near the coast at Coumeenole Beach. During the summer, while Méiní's son Séamus was living in the old house on the Blaskets, Martin lived with Méiní in her little house, returning to his own place when Séamus was on the mainland.

Some time at the beginning of January 1955, Martin brought me to meet his old aunt in her cottage. He had warned me that she smoked a pipe, so I armed myself with some plug tobacco and a small bottle of whiskey as an introductory present. The cottage that I entered was very small and consisted of a single room. Two beds stood end to end on the right-hand side as you entered the half-door, with a small loft overhead. To the left of the doorway was a tiny window flanked by a rough deal table. Further left in the gable wall was a tiny turf fire on a level with the floor. Instead of the wooden or metal crane over the fire which was common in such houses on the mainland and on the island, and which enabled the kettle or the cooking-pot to be adjusted in its height above the fire, there was a rudimentary hanger attached to the wall, in shape like a tongs, with two hooks at its lower ends. Méiní sat on a tiny stool beside the fire, near enough to tend the pot without having to get up from a sitting position. One or two rather greasy rope chairs stood on the earthen floor. Opposite the half-door a small window looked out over the islands.

The setting was one of extreme discomfort and apparent poverty, but two factors transformed it. The house was warm and in midwinter one could appreciate this as one came from the cold outside. There were draughts, of course, but owing to the fact that the fire was literally never out and because the walls were thick, there was a feeling of dryness and comfort which belied the Spartan surroundings. In the second place, the little room radiated with the warmth of Méiní's welcome and sense of humour. On this first occasion, the pipe was crammed with the tobacco I had brought, and lit from the fire; the bottle of whiskey was lovingly caressed. My strange Christian name Méiní was never to master. *Italy* was the nearest she could get to it and Italy it was to remain. She held the little bottle up before my face and with an infectious twinkle in her eyes she said it for the first of many times in Irish: 'Italy, my boy, tonight I'll be stretched out on the bed with this bottle, and me ass will be high in the air!'

Martin was as interested as Méiní in telling tales of traditional types and in swopping stories of their ancestors or people they had known in their youth. To Méiní's Blasket stories Martin could add his own, which he had collected as far east as Castlemaine, at the head of the peninsula, where he had worked as a young man. After my first introduction,

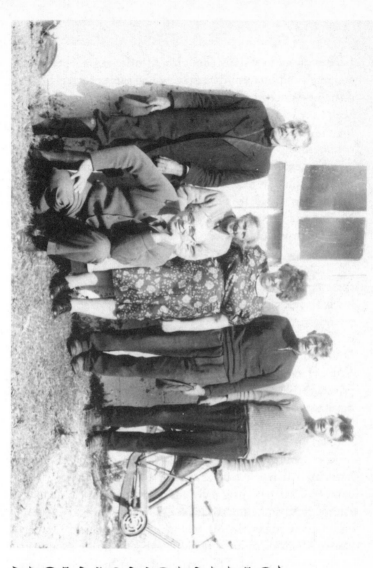

At Ballinarabha, 1962
(Standing, left to
right)
Eoghan Sheáin
Eoghain (Méiní's
elder stepson), Méiní
Máire Kilcoyne
(Méiní's daughter),
Séamus (Méiní's son
and Eoghan Mór Ó
Catháin (her
nephew, an
accomplished sean-
nós singer)
(In front) Austin
Kilcoyne, Máire's
husband

I never went to visit Méiní without bringing a notebook, and rarely did I return without recording some proverb, riddle or tale produced by Martin or herself. She was particularly keen to tell me the story of her life and her obvious nostalgia for the Blaskets was evident in the stories she told of that community.

The next summer I returned again and Martin brought me immediately to Méiní. The reaction was the same as before. She loved to sit with her back towards the ditch, Martin and myself crouched at her side. As she talked she would occasionally translate some tricky phrase into English, or Martin would supply a gloss. Then everything would break off while her gnarled hands played with the pipe, pushing the smouldering tobacco further down the bowl with her index finger, which was entirely black and scarred from this operation.

The next year brought a major talking-point to the Dunquin community – the granting of the drink licence to Kruger Kavanagh in spite of the opposition of the local parish priest, Father Tom Moriarty. At about the same time, Peig Sayer's son Mike was appointed a collector for the Irish Folklore Commission. For the next few years he came regularly to Méiní to take down her stories, now available in his own hand in the archives of the commission. He himself has stated that what he sent to the commission were fair copies of what he originally took down in his notebooks. Although in some instances he has been known to exercise a certain creativity in his treatment of his sources, in the case of Méiní's account of her life there is no reason to suspect anything of the sort. The flavour of what he has preserved for us has the authentic Méiní touch which matches well what others have recorded.

In 1958, Peig Sayers, to whom Méiní had been such a comfort in her time of grief, died in Dingle hospital. Since her return to Dunquin in 1942 she had seen little of Méiní, and for some years before her death she had been in the hospital, her sight rapidly fading. As there were only three or four years between them, Peig's death brought home to Méiní the realisation that her own time was short. She always spoke of the sadness of Peig's life – the sudden loss of her son, her separation from her exiled family. Merciful providence concealed from Méiní that in the next few years almost unrelieved sadness was to be her own lot.

In early 1961, her nephew Martin moved into the County Home in Killarney and was to stay there for the next three years. That July, I set off for Dunquin in my first car, calling on him on my journey. My first thought on arriving at Dunquin was to persuade Méiní, who was now, by my reckoning, eighty-five years of age, to come on a tour of exploration of Murreagh, Feohanagh and Ballydavid, to the north of the peninsula. Though her stories were full of references to Kilmalkedar parish and the 'Parish o' Moore' in which these places were to be found, it was the first time that she had visited them. The furthest point to which our journey took us was seven miles as the crow flies from Dunquin, but her excitement could hardly have been exceeded if she was on a world tour. The harbour at Baile na nGall, misnamed Ballydavid by the coastguards the century before, was inspected from the car with the knowing eye of a fisherman's widow. One might have thought that to someone like Méiní, who had been born in the United States and had crossed the Atlantic three times, such sights would have provided little interest. Far from it. She returned to her cottage tired but blissfully happy as a result of all she had seen.

In the summer of 1962, Méiní's daughter Máire came on a visit with her husband Austin Kilcoyne and she stayed in the house in Ballinaraha which Séamus her brother shared with two other former Blasket men. For the duration of this visit, Méiní moved up to that house to be with her family.

My wife and I visited the group at Ballinaraha on an occasion when there was a gathering of Blasket people. Kate Pheats Tom Ní Cheárnaigh was home on a visit from America and brought her mother 'Nelly Jerry' to visit. Lisa Mistéal of Carhoo, a niece of the 'Lís Daly who was the companion to Méiní on her trip to the United States, was also there.

Before the summer was out, having borrowed a tape recorder, I persuaded Méiní and Máire to make a recording. On 4 September we made the journey to Kruger's Guest House where electricity had been installed, and made the recording in a bedroom there. Méiní's hearing had greatly deteriorated by this stage and she did not always grasp the instructions Máire gave her in relation to timing. Nevertheless, she told a few stories and talked about her early life before giving up exhausted after about twenty minutes. When in full flight, her obvious enthusiasm for what she was telling us belied her eighty-six years.

The year 1963 was to prove a lonely and a tragic one for Méiní. There was little news from Martin, who before he went to Killarney had been spending more and more time with her and sharing her house while Séamus was away fishing. At the beginning of the year, Lisa Mistéal sent a report: 'Poor old Méiní is holding her own. The poor soul. I saw her last week. No change. The same as ever. But the winter is very long. God bless her.'

In the month of February, Lisa reported on the severe winter: 'We never saw any winter as bad – since Christmas it was terrible. Plenty of frost for a few weeks and blowing hard. Then followed an ominous detail: 'Séamus was not so well there for a couple of weeks . . . he had a corn on his toe and it was terribly sore. He is fine now. When he gets a cold or anything it takes a lot out of him. Méiní is the best and she so old. Gets up every day and no change.'

In July, the news about Séamus was bad, as Lisa reported: 'I was down to see Méiní last night and honestly I could cry for her. Poor Séamus is bad and I believe his second toe will be taken off. He had a terrible pain and he went to the doctor and he ordered him to the Dingle Hospital and after a few days he was shifted to Tralee.' Apparently something more serious than a corn was in question.

Méiní's interest in babies was not diminishing and after my marriage in 1961 she never ceased to enquire about the cradle. In that July letter, Lisa told of her reaction to the news she brought: 'Poor Méiní asked me if I had heard from you, and I said "Yes," and she pulled me closer to her and asked me for sure and certain about the cradle. "With the help of God," I said, and she was so glad the poor soul. I brought her a few homemade buns just like homemade bread. God help her, I felt sorry for her. The poor soul is all alone now. Only for Bobby, he stays with her while Séamus is away. She is so anxious to see him back.'

During that summer of 1963, Séamus was continually under treatment for his poisoned foot, but on 2 September he returned back in Kruger's van to Dunquin. The nearest point of the road to Méiní's house was just outside Máirín Sheehy's house in Ballykeen. Getting out of the van, he collapsed, but with the help of his cousin Bobby, he got up before falling again. Dr Séamus McEntee, who happened to be walking by with his wife, helped Bobby, now joined by Méiní's grandnephew Tomás, to bring Séamus down to his own house. He had got as far as the gate when he collapsed and died. Méiní was taking her tea when Bobby came in to get a chair with which to lift the dead man but when they brought him in his mother did not recognise him and asked what had happened to the stranger. They broke the sad news to her then. According to Lisa, Méiní bore up remarkably well under this cruel blow but was particularly distressed that with the local phone broken down, immediate word could not be sent to her daughter Máire in Springfield. It may be that she felt the news would bring Máire home again, though it was less than a year since her last visit.

Séamus was buried in the new graveyard which looked down over the Blaskets between Dunquin and Coumeenole. As the autumn days lengthened into winter his mother's spirit was sorely tried. Bobby moved up permanently from the Muileann to care for his aunt, and her grandnephew Tomás also did his share in minding her. He enjoyed her company and his comings and goings kept her spirits from collapsing altogether. The month after Séamus's death, Méiní's prayers were answered and my wife gave birth to our first daughter. Lisa brought her the news and reported her delight. November brought news of the death of her former employer, the ex-teacher Dan Lynch.

Méiní's spirits received a lift the following July when her nephew Martin Keane returned after his years in the County Home in Killarney. From my visits to him I had been able to bring some news to Dunquin, but that was at long intervals. Now he immediately took over the job of looking after Méiní and slept in the bed which was head to toe with her own. Bobby went back to the house at the Muileann which he had shared with Martin and their brother Billy who had died seven years before. Although Martin ragged her from time to time and on occasion dismissed her comments very abrasively, there was real companionship between them. Martin's laborious trips on his crutches to have a drink at Kruger's pub enabled him to bring back news of the wider world. In the tourist season there were occasional visitors to the cottage, attracted by Méiní's reputation as a character, and Mike Pheig Sayers kept up his visits to glean her full repertoire of stories. I was able to keep in touch with Méiní and Martin between my visits, because their neighbour Mrs Máirín Sheehy wrote to me on Martin's behalf. Méiní's delight in having Martin back with her was crowned in the same summer by another visit from her beloved Máire, a year after her brother's death.

On my trips I found it was becoming harder and harder to persuade Méiní to leave her cottage. When the weather was fine she would come out and lean against the ditch in front of her gate. When she was unable to come out, Martin and I would go down to Béal Átha where the old mill had been. One tiny field there was called the Forge Garden and there in Garraí na Ceartan Martin and I would sit watching the crane, carrying her usual nickname of 'Junie an Scrogaill', or the two white swans that would occasionally visit there, to Martin's delight. In the last days of 1964 Máirín Sheehy again wrote on Martin's behalf saying how much he was looking forward to giving me more Irish lessons at the Forge Garden school in the following summer.

In August 1965, Joan and I took our daughter Kristin, now a few weeks short of her second birthday, to visit Méiní. As the old woman fondled the child, Martin and I slipped off to the Forge Garden to take down another story in Irish; two days later he told me, and I wrote down, a story from the Finn cycle which was to be his last story for me. Twelve days before Christmas, while still living in Méiní's house, he collapsed across his bed and died. Méiní was in bed herself and was unable to summon help. Of her many nephews, Martin had been the closest to her; the blow tested her resilient spirit to its limits.

Again the extended family rallied around. Bobby once more moved up to Méiní's house to resume caring for her, a task which Martin had performed since his return home. This arrangement was to last for little more than a year; the reaper had not yet finished his labour. In early February, 1967, Bobby himself fell ill and was moved to hospital. He lived for one week only and was brought back to Dunquin for burial. 'God help her,' wrote Lisa Mistéal. 'She is a pity now! I went to see Bobby in hospital, he was terribly thirsty and I knew he was going to die. They are all gone now. Billy, Séamus, poor Martin and now Tomás (Bobby's real name) is gone. I was down Sunday evening, and honestly Méiní could get you very upset. Now the other house is empty. I mean the house Méiní used to live in. God help them, they were a quiet family.'

Immediately after Bobby's death, as Lisa had written, Méiní moved a couple of hundred yards into one of the houses at the Muileann above Béal Átha in which another of her nephews, Michael Keane, known as 'Noden', lived with his son Tomás. Although the house was tiny, it was beside that which had been earlier occupied by Martin, Billy and Bobby, and this gave extra space. Michael's wife Nell Gromell had died ten years before, and he and his son looked after Méiní with the occasional help of neighbours such as Mrs Máirín Sheehy. But it was not to be for long. She was now in extreme old age, over ninety, and the previous four years of deep personal bereavement had exacted a heavy toll.

In the early hours of Sunday, 23 April 1967, the struggle was over, and Méiní joined Seán Eoghain, Séamus, Martin and the others on the 'way of truth'. In the final weeks she had been sinking fast. Lisa Mistéal had visited her on the Sunday before her death, and noticed a big decline: 'She wasn't like herself at all – kind of restless. Oh, I felt so sorry for her.' Going into Mass that Sunday morning, Lisa met 'Piley' Moriarty, who told her the news. Maurice Moriarty, a brother of Kate, was one of Méiní's nearest neighbours, and lived a few yards down the hill from Máirín Sheehy.

On Monday 24 April, Méiní was buried, as Séamus had been, in the new cemetery which enclosed land which had once belonged to the Sheehy family. Though she now rested in what she always looked upon as her home parish, it was fitting that her grave faced over the Blasket Islands which she had loved so well and where the best years of her life had been passed.

As Méiní lay in her bed, feeling life ebbing away from her and her grip on time becoming looser, ever looser, the preoccupations of daily life slipped further and further from her mind. We can but guess that her thoughts travelled back, further and still further through the events and impressions of her long life, blending together, swirling like the falling leaves of autumn. She could see Martin collapsed on his bed, Máire waving goodbye from the motor-car and Séamus slumped in death on her old rope chair. By candlelight, Italy wrote in his notebook at the table by the half-door; there was Dan Lynch's cow waiting to be milked and her old mother welcoming her back from the island. As the cock crew, there was Seán Eoghain stretched out, and yet again Peig kneeling in despairing prayer before the statue of the Virgin. And now the flashing of Father Griffin's eyes, and Pat Casht playing his fiddle and Séamus lying in his cradle. Yes, there was Dr Hudson standing with his pipe; now he is lying down with Peggy Flint's needle in his backside. And again Seán Eoghain trembling because of the cat under the bed; now he is setting out from the Blaskets in his *naomhóg* on the dawn of their wedding-day. The *Majestic* is sailing into Cork Harbour and Jimmy Hickey is beside her in the train. And 'Lís Daly is laughing at her seasick friend, and she can smell the whetstone oil clinging to her hair. Now here is Kate coming down the Clasach road with a load of turf; on the Commons of Ballykeen old Keating's donkey is grazing. Far, far back, there is her grandfather bending over his loom and farthest away of all the lank grass in the lonely cemetery at Chicopee.

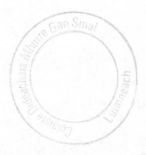